AF785057

Harv—

So like, when are we doing one of these on you.—

Bill

November 1993

A smile is the beginning.

Operation Smile
INTERNATIONAL

the first ten years

P U B L I S H E R

Operation Smile International

717 Boush Street Norfolk, Virginia 23510 United States of America 804 625 0375

P H O T O G R A P H Y

Mark Edward Atkinson

unless otherwise noted

P H O T O G R A P H I C P R I N T S

Joseph A. Mishkofski

B O O K D E S I G N

William L. Owen, Jr.

P R I N T E R

Direct Printing Company, LTD.

printed in Hong Kong

for underwriting color separations, we thank

Hutchison Whampoa Limited

for underwriting book bindery, we thank

Operation Smile China Medical Mission Limited

Copyright: Operation Smile International
All rights reserved.

ISBN 0-9635271-0-X

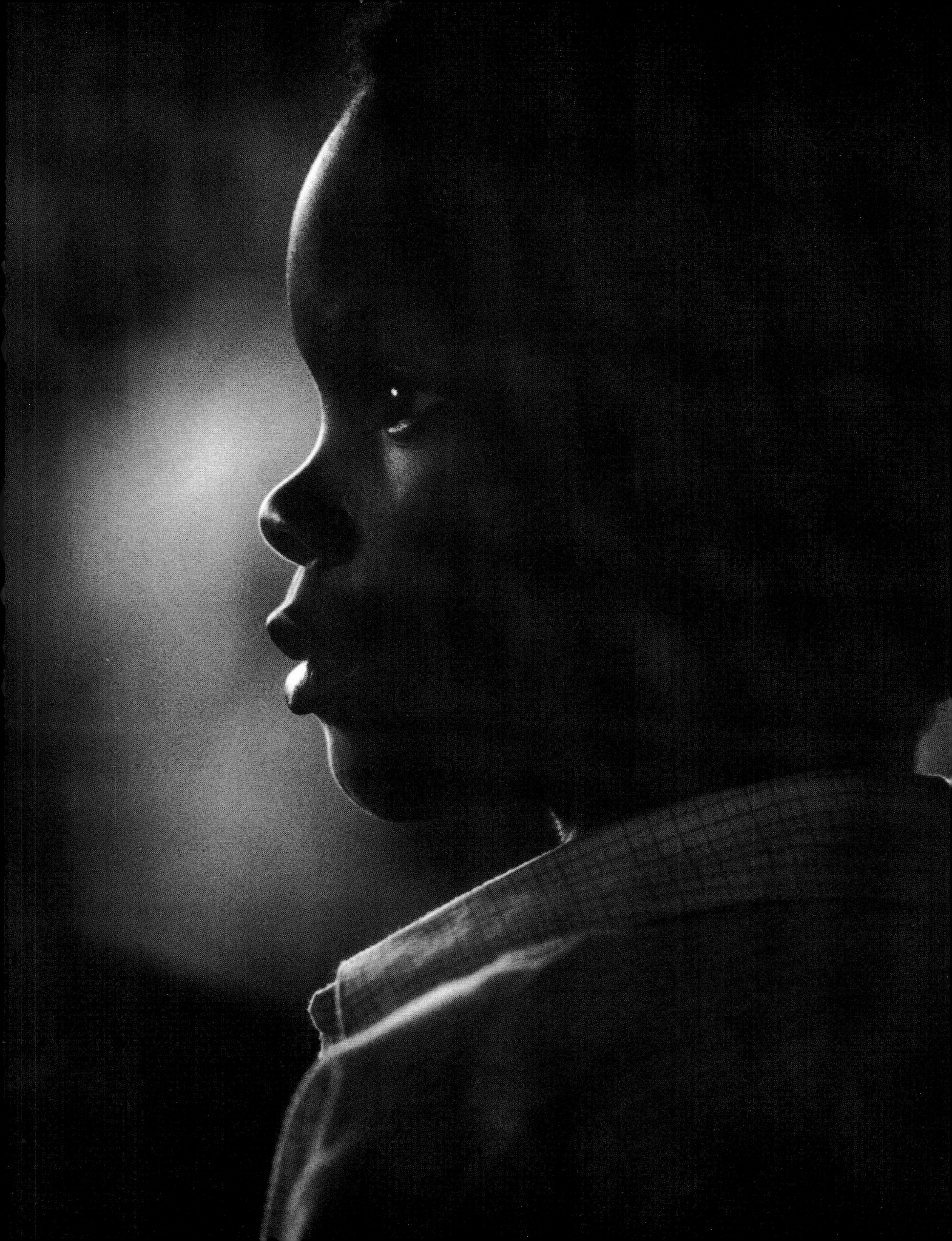

DEDICATION

John Connor devotedly gave of himself to our mission
of caring for the children of the world.
In his spirit, and to the spirit of our volunteers, we dedicate this book.

Founded in 1982 by Bill and Kathy Magee, Operation Smile International is a private, nonprofit medical/educational organization providing reconstructive surgery and related healthcare to indigent children and young adults in developing countries and the United States.

May the inspiring example of your witness of God's care and love continue to grow and draw others to do the same.

MOTHER TERESA
MISSION OF CHARITIES

Since 1982 Operation Smile has taken our family on a journey around the world. The pictures embedded in our hearts and minds, in our very souls, each have stories we may never get to tell. However, these pictures tell a different story to each viewer, each important, each potentially life-changing. The thousands of wonderful people who have walked by our side are the ones who have made the difference. They have shared the experiences, felt the gripping pain and tears that are shed when we cannot help someone for lack of supplies, time, or ability. They have also had the privilege of feeling the immeasurable joy of watching a child's transformation from a life of shame and disfigurement to a life of joy and happiness. Imagine a mother or father who just days before was tugging on your sleeve, literally begging you to help their child, days later bonding with you as a brother or sister of our world. That family member and you shared only one common link in the beginning — you both wanted their child to be able to live a normal life. Both took risks. You, the volunteer, by entering into an unknown region of the world and they, taking the biggest risk, trusting the life of their child to a stranger. Both parties experienced joy in those events. And because of it, both become better citizens of the world.

In a world of increasing complexity our challenge is to find and hold tightly the simplest of truths; that life is a mirror, and how we live will be reflected back to us. The simple truth is that we all have a need to love and to be loved. These are important as we strive for fulfillment. Our simple truth is that since 1982 tens of thousands of children in the U.S.A. and in developing countries have begun a new life because of the generosity of tens of thousands of volunteers who have shared their time, talents, and treasures. The simple truth is that we all know when we are doing something right or wrong. When we see a child in need, when we kneel down to help that child and their family begin a new life, we are doing the work that God meant us to do when he gave us the privilege to inhabit this earth. This book is a tribute to those efforts.

Thank you for being at our side.

Bill and Kathy Magee

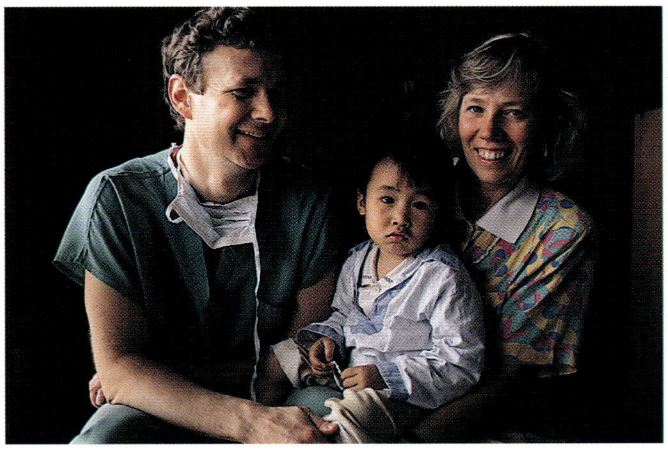

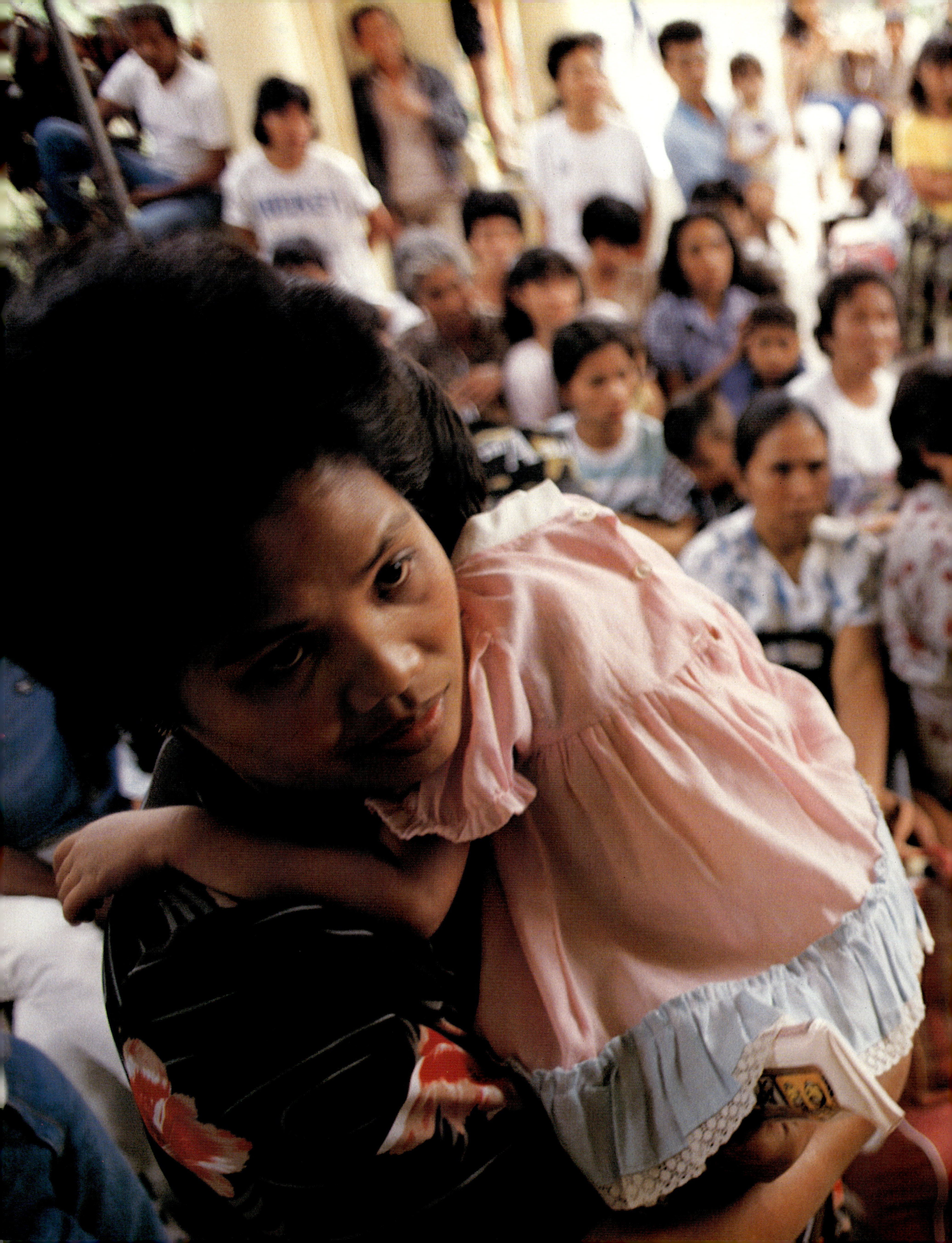

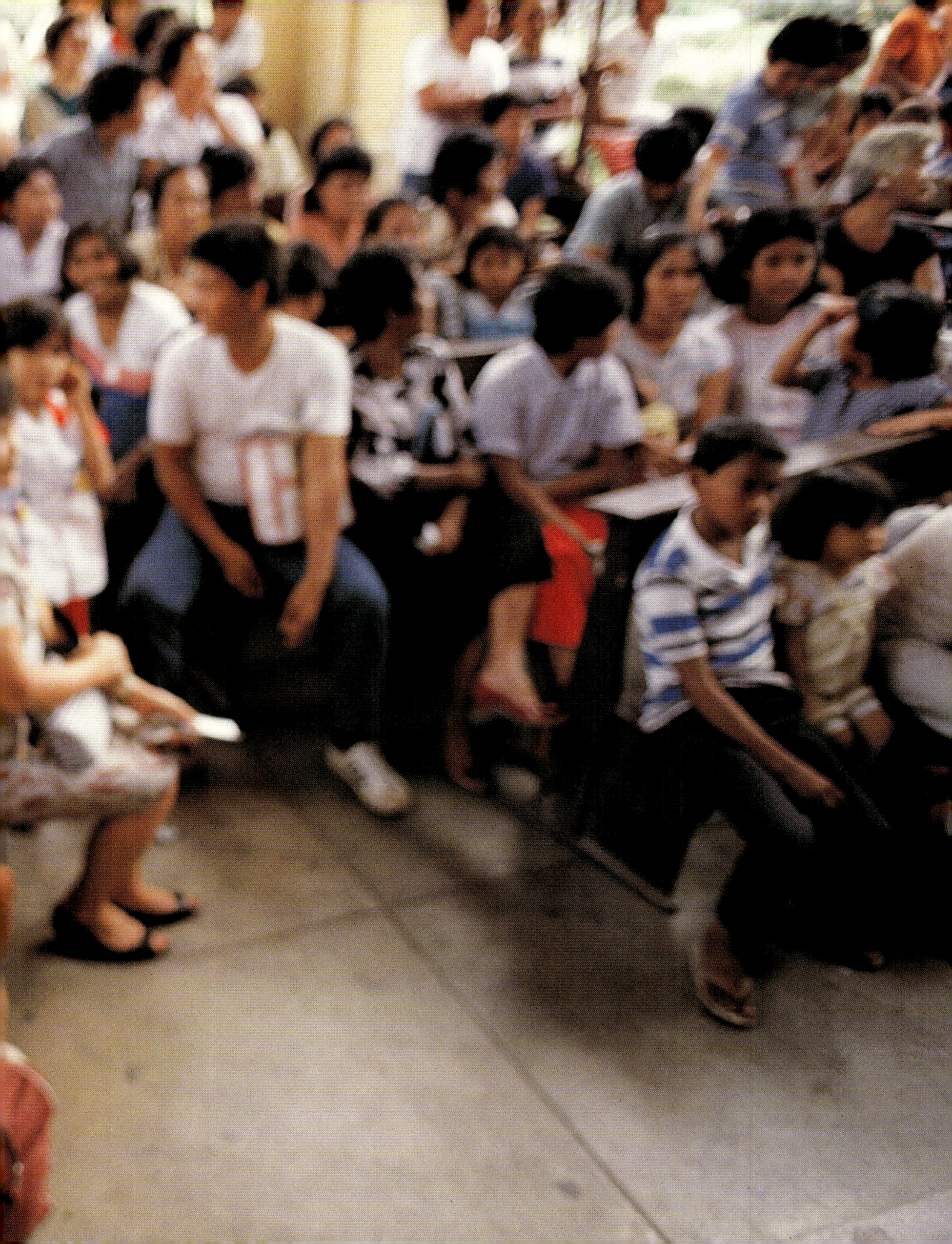

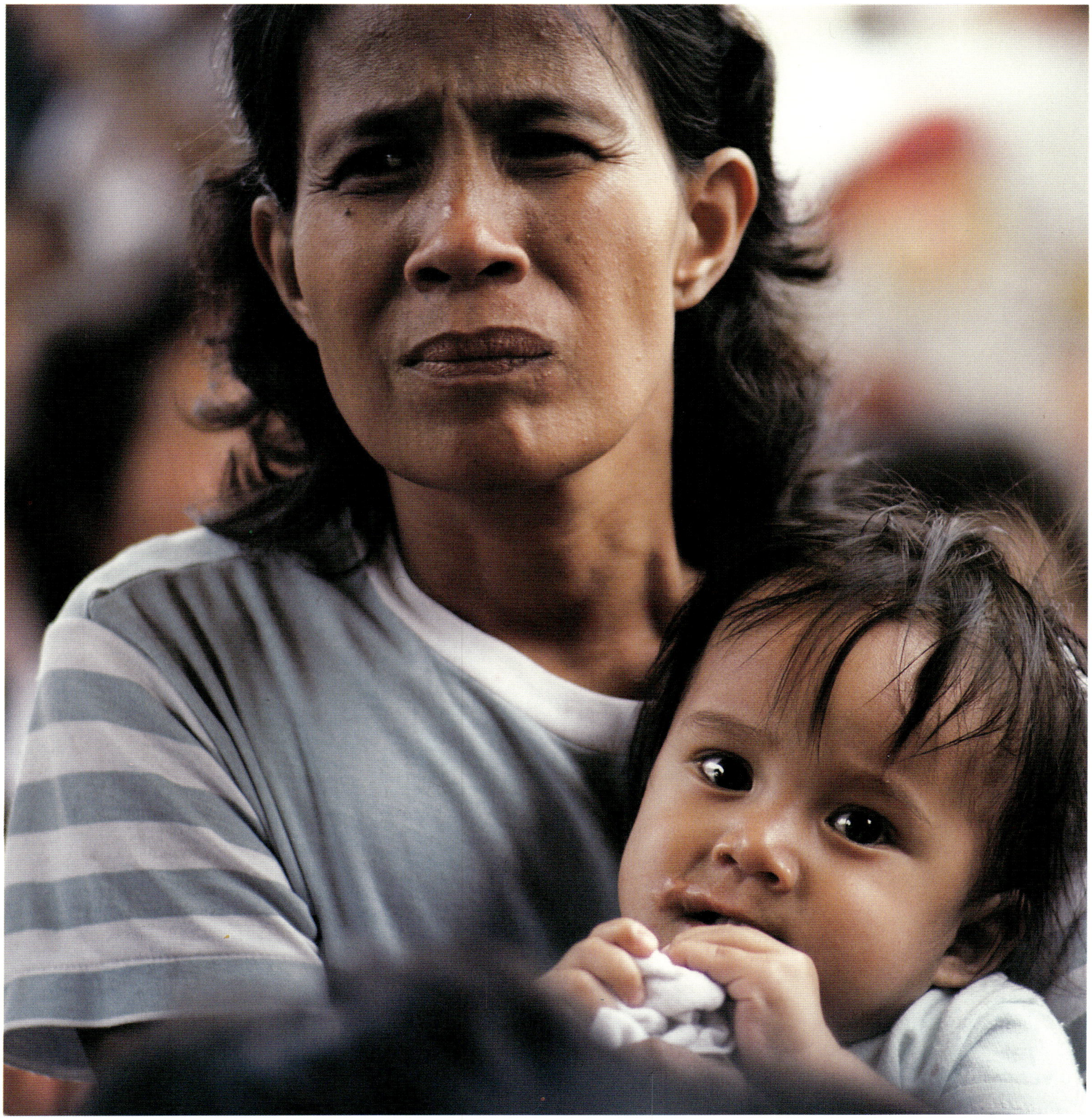

mother and child, Naga City
(previous page) families wait for screening, Naga City

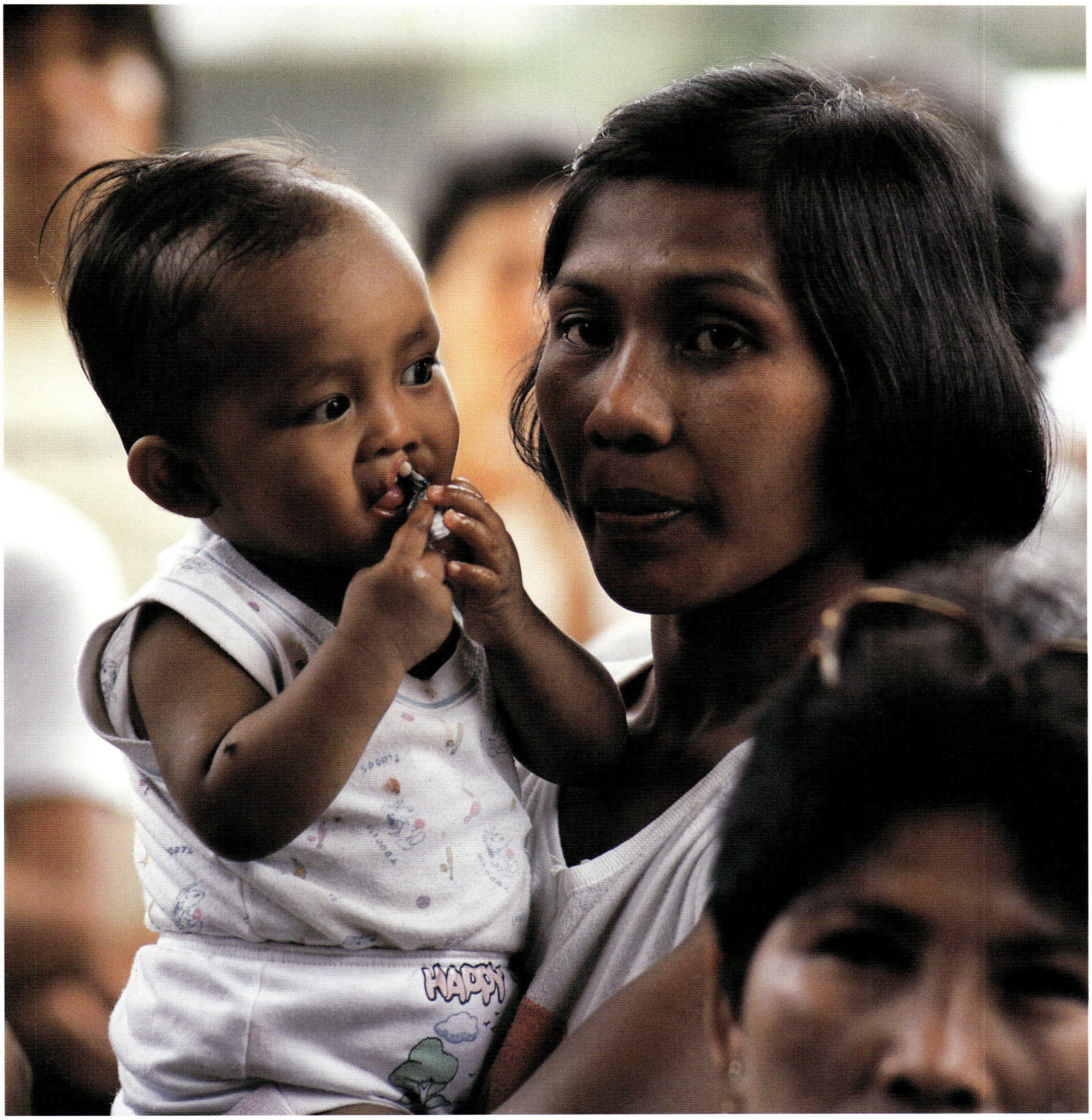

mother and child, Naga City

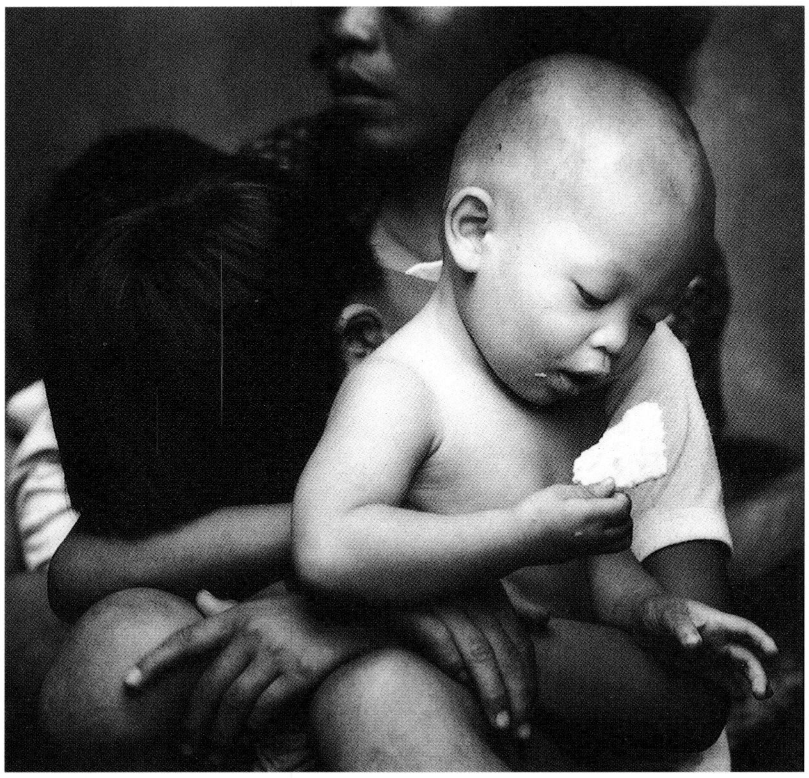

patients, Manila

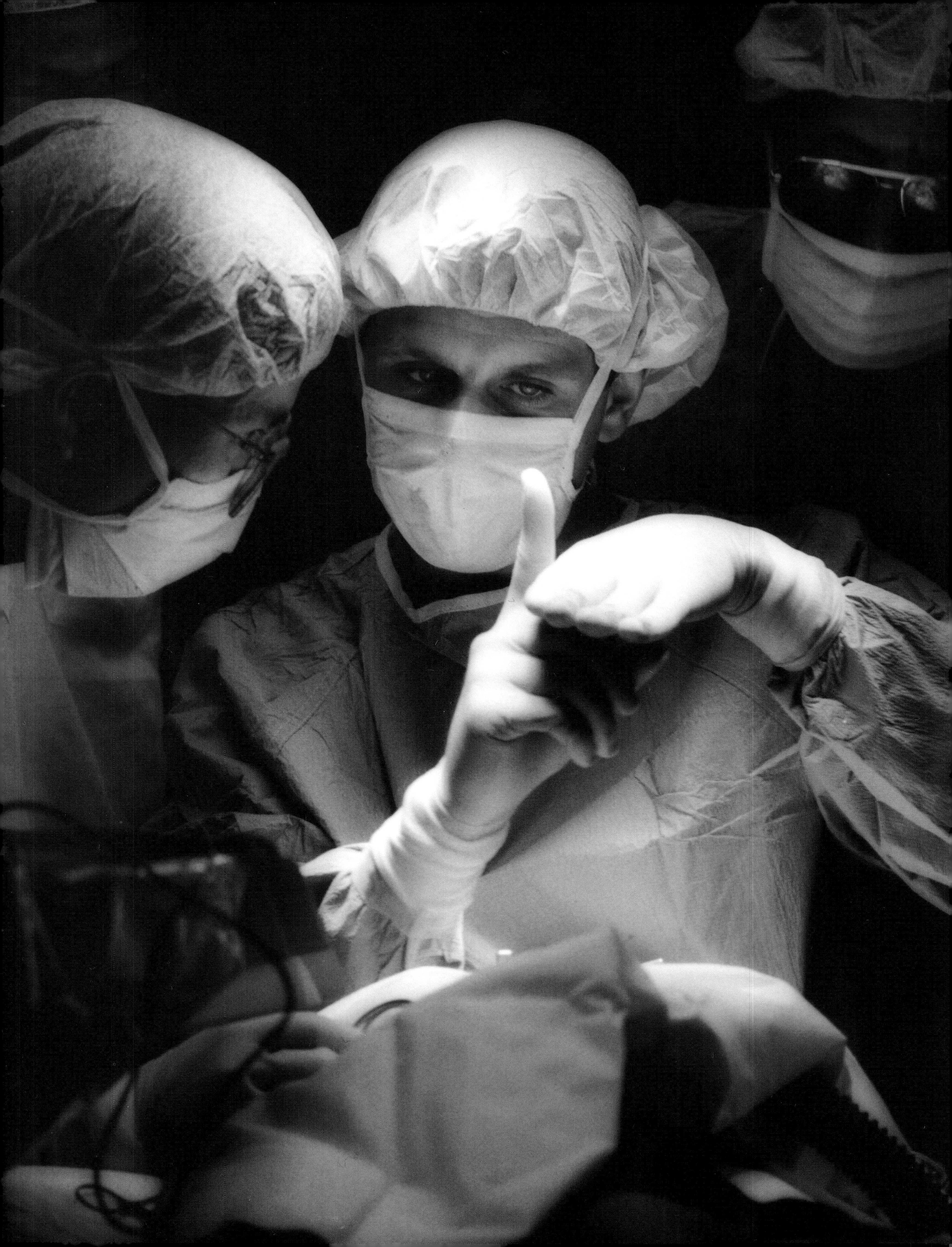

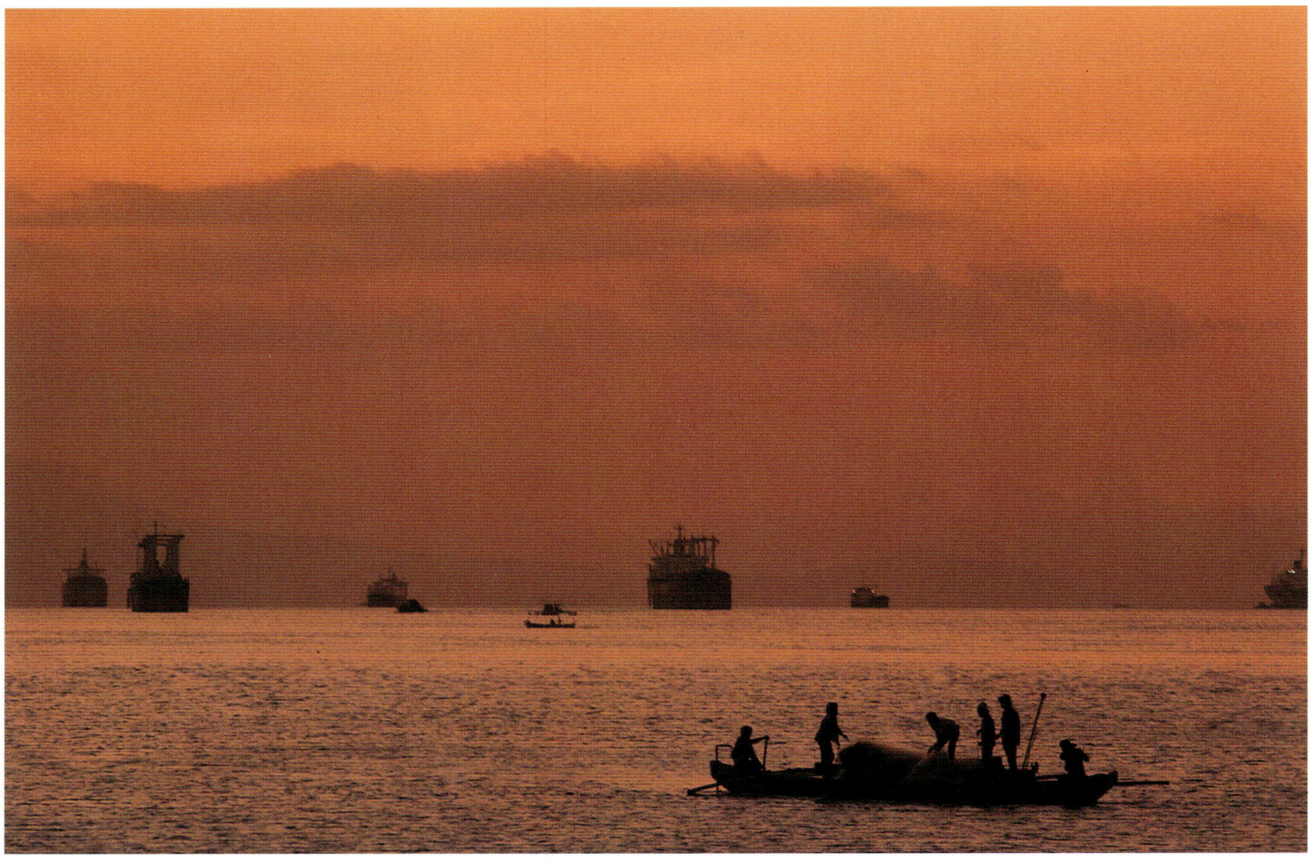

ships and fishermen, Manila Bay

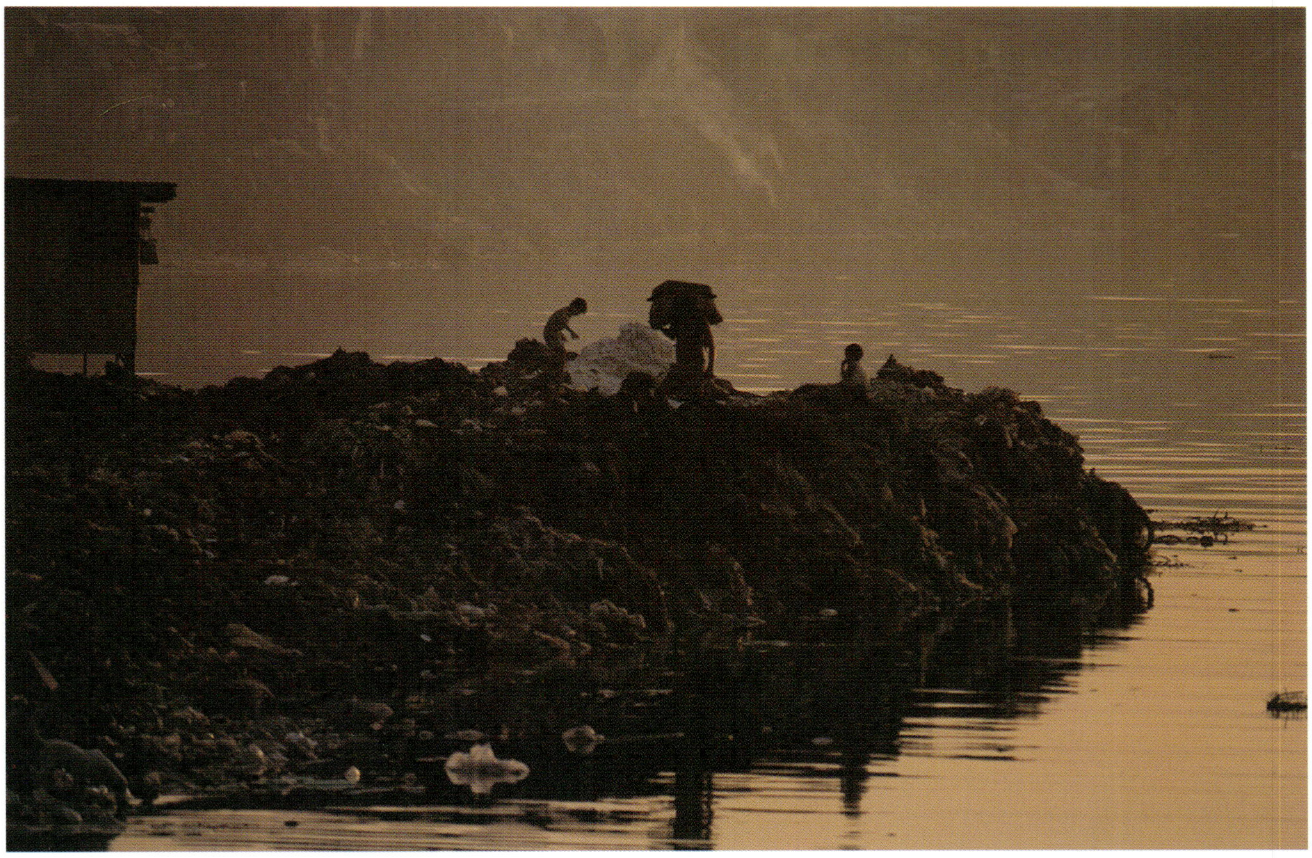

children, metro Manila dump

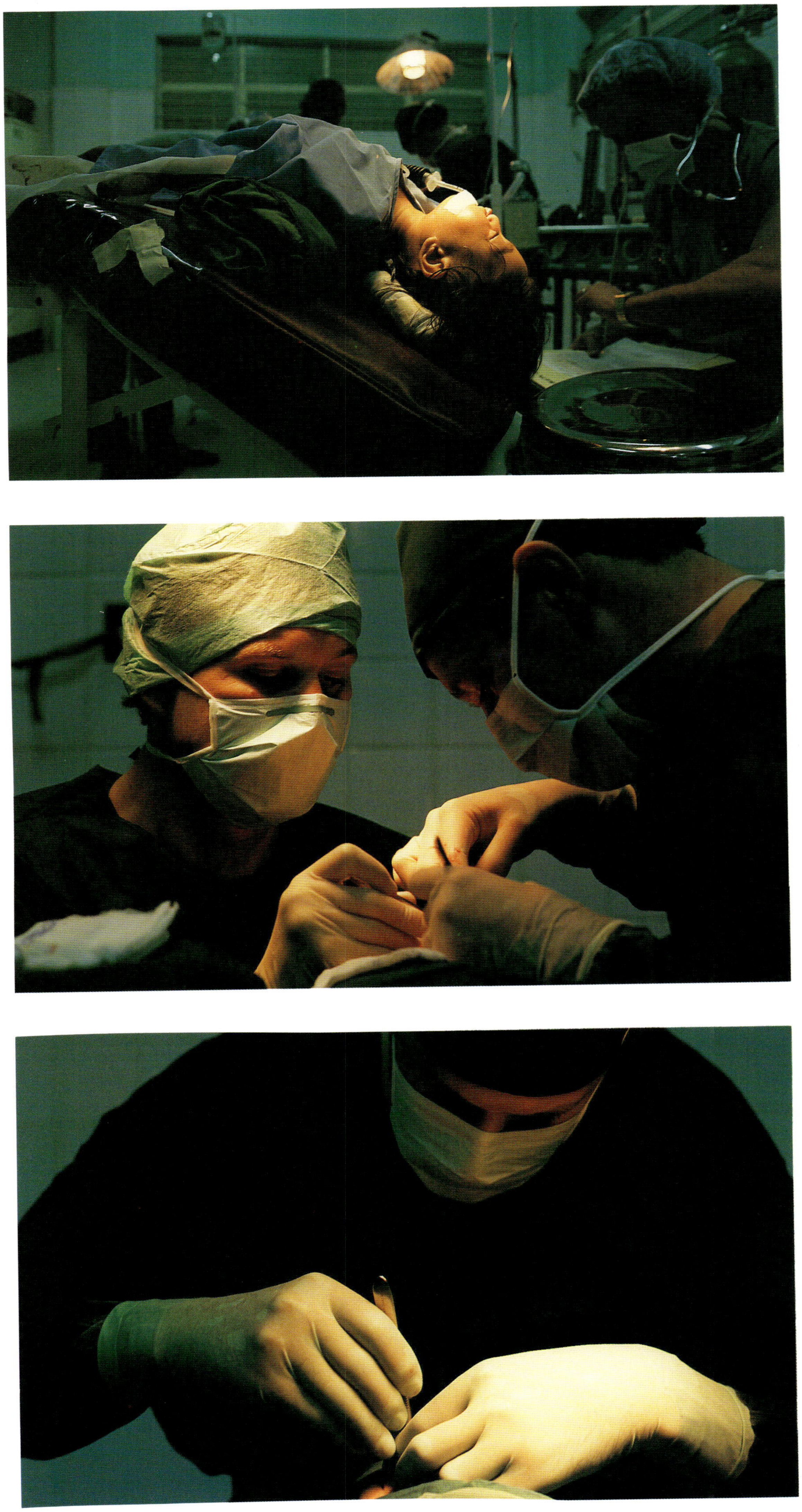

surgery, Naga City

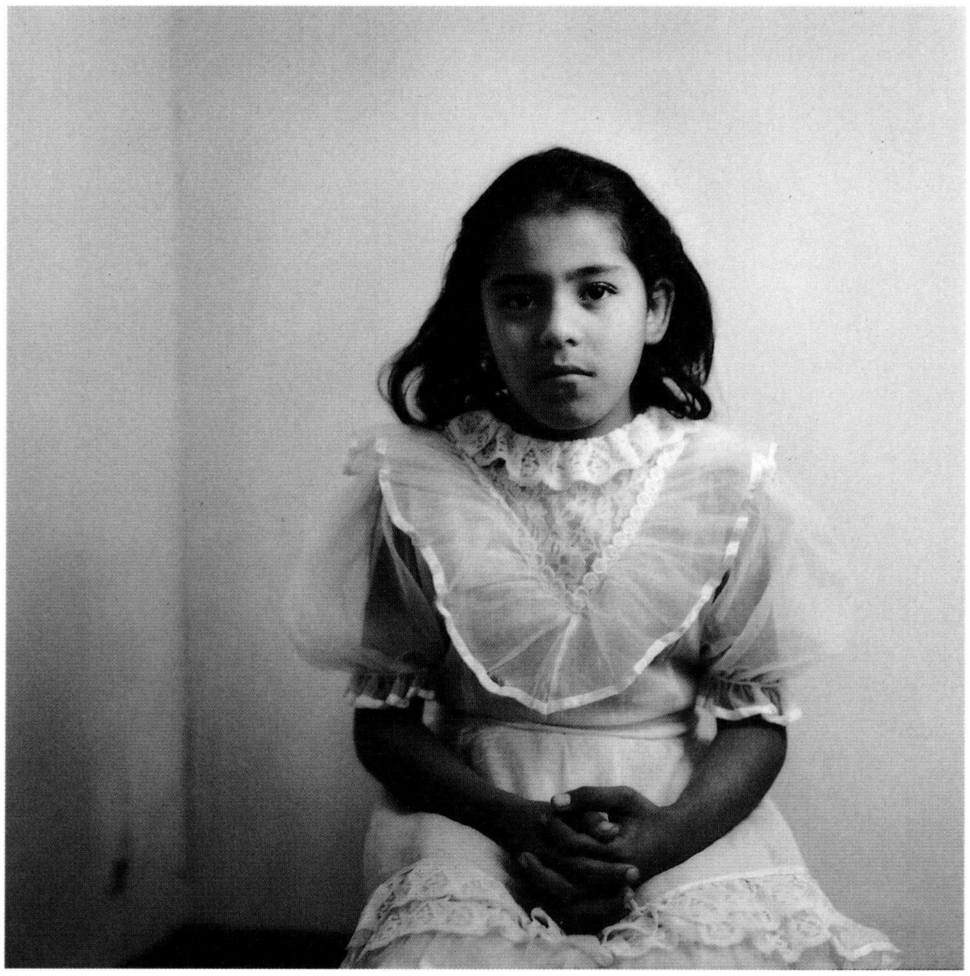

patient, Colombian peasant girl

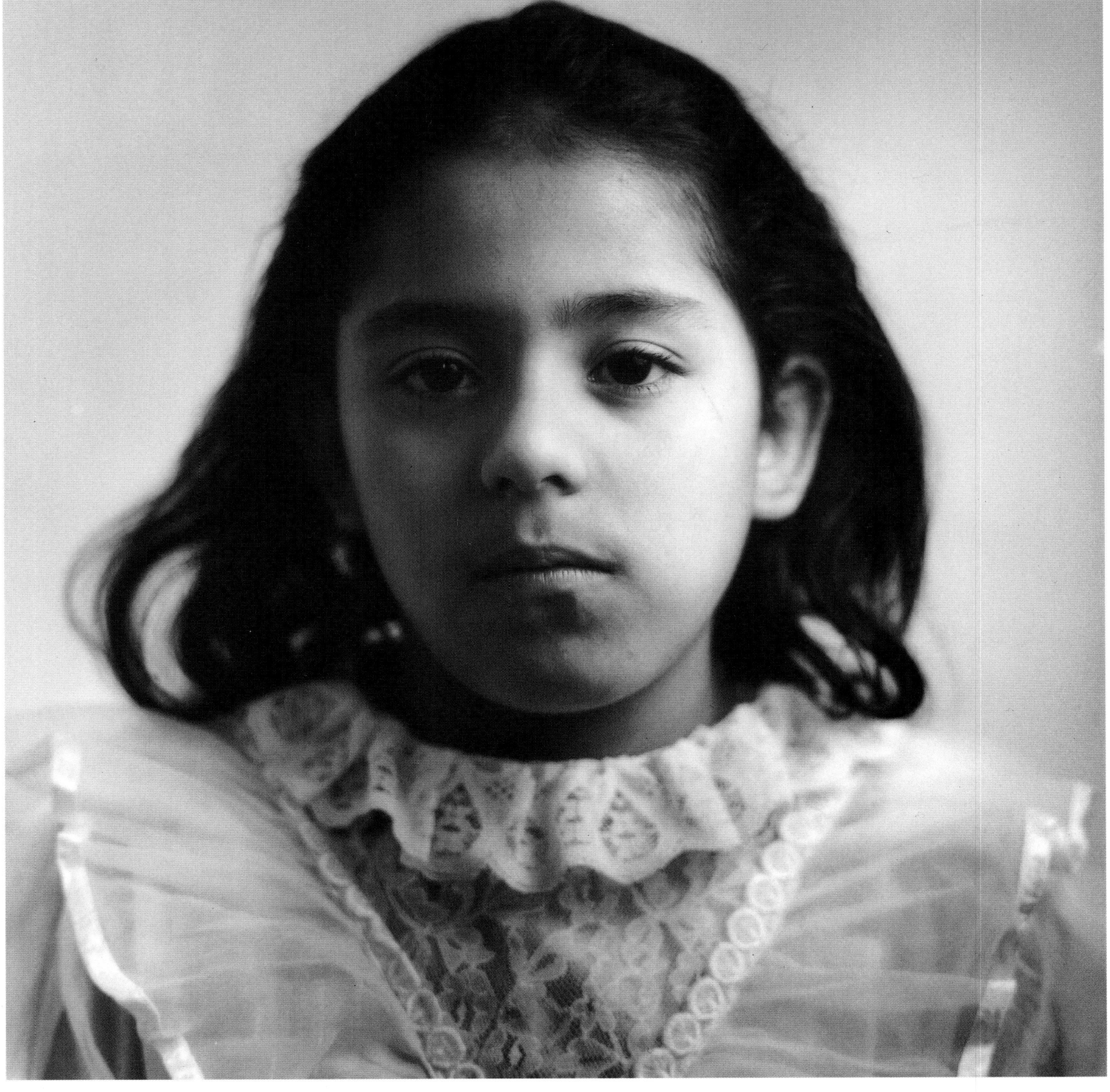

*These children were strong beyond all telling of strength,
they were brave against all odds.*

KATIE BERGIN
OSI YOUTH CLUB VOLUNTEER

mother and child, Hangzhou

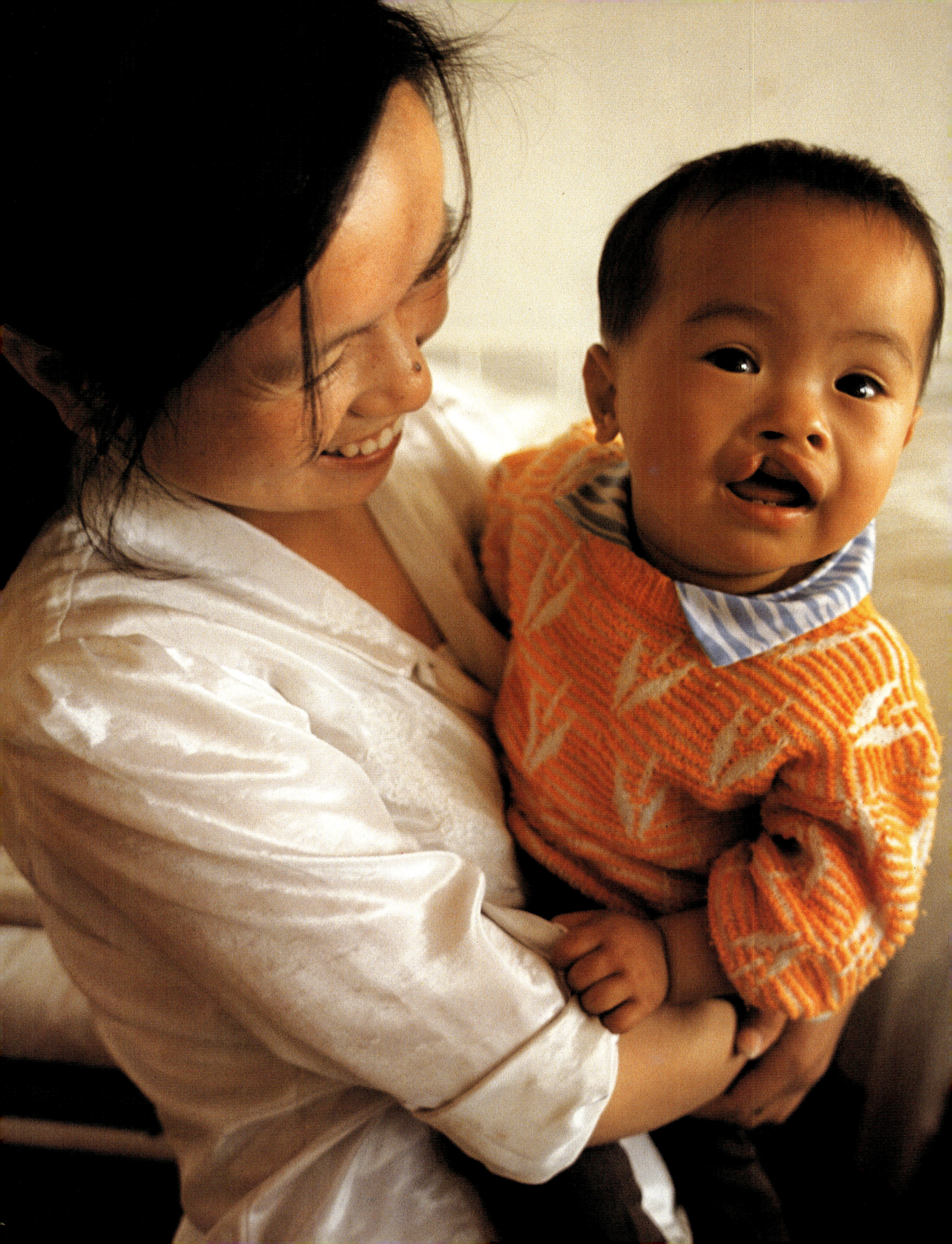

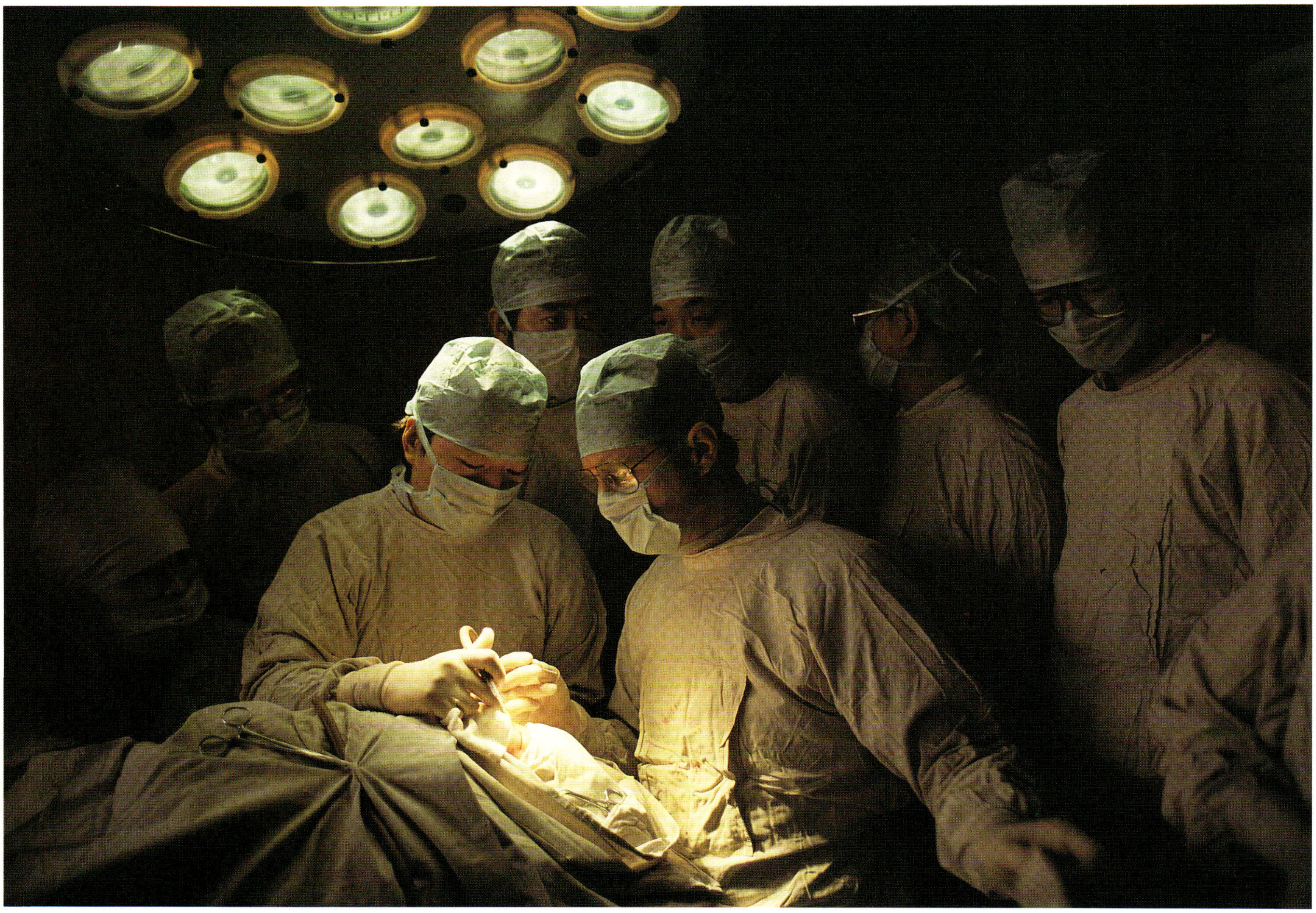

surgery, Hangzhou

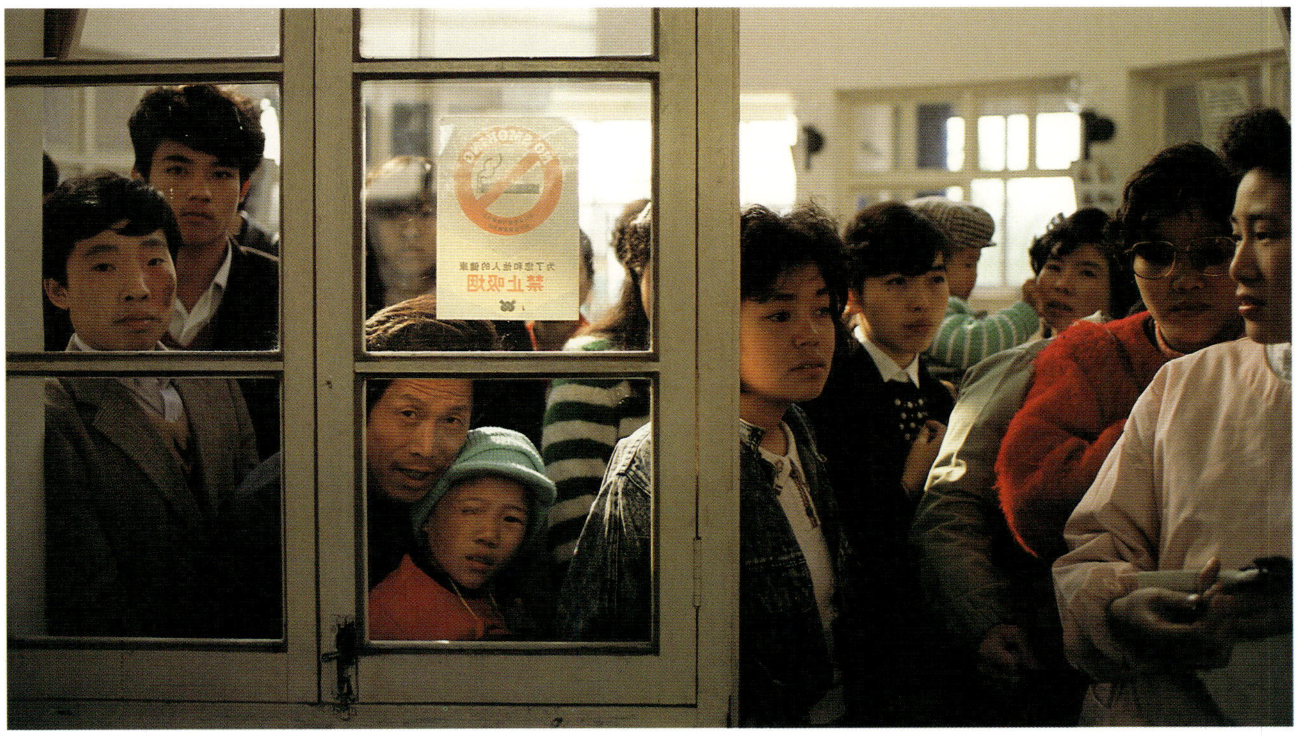

screening, Hangzhou

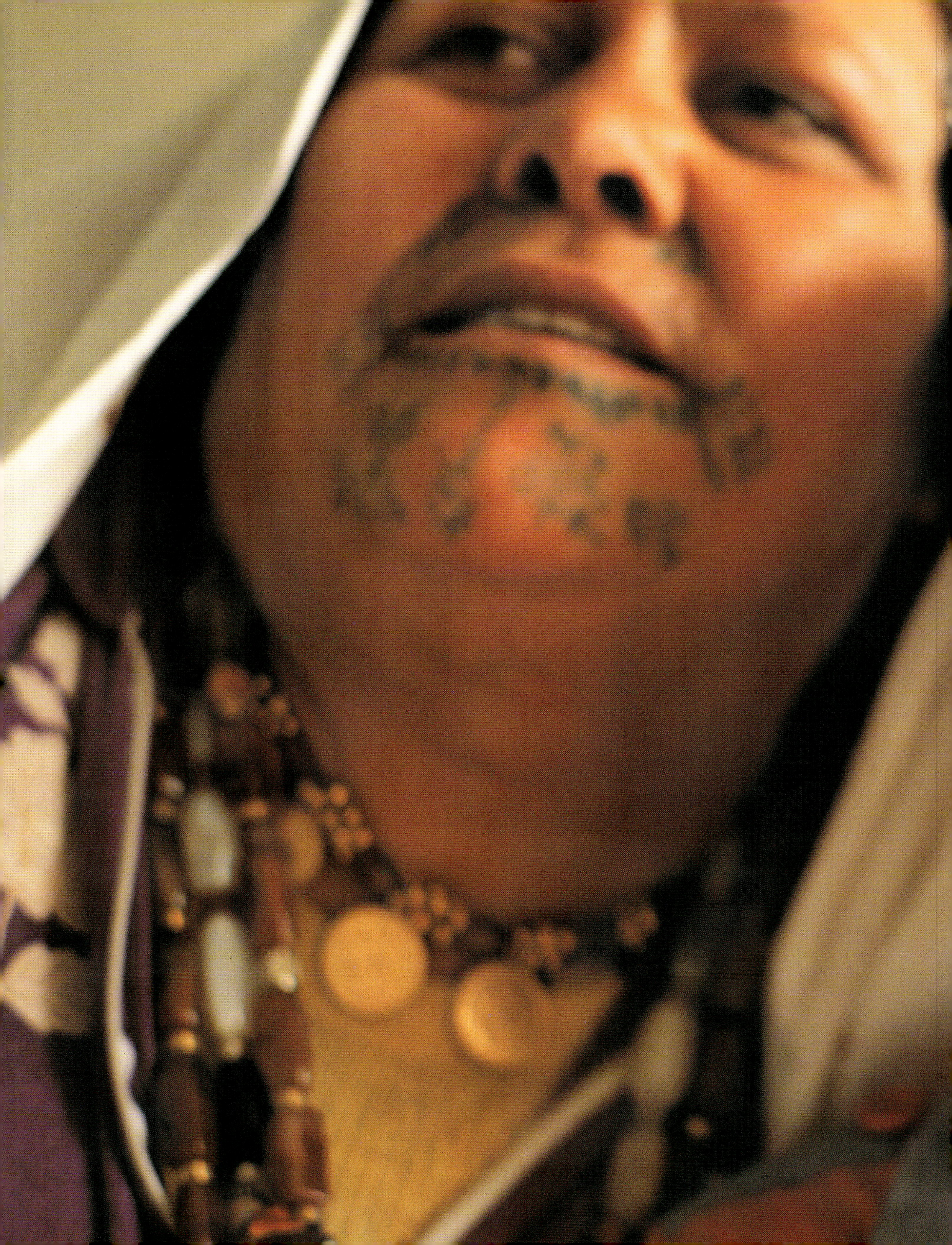

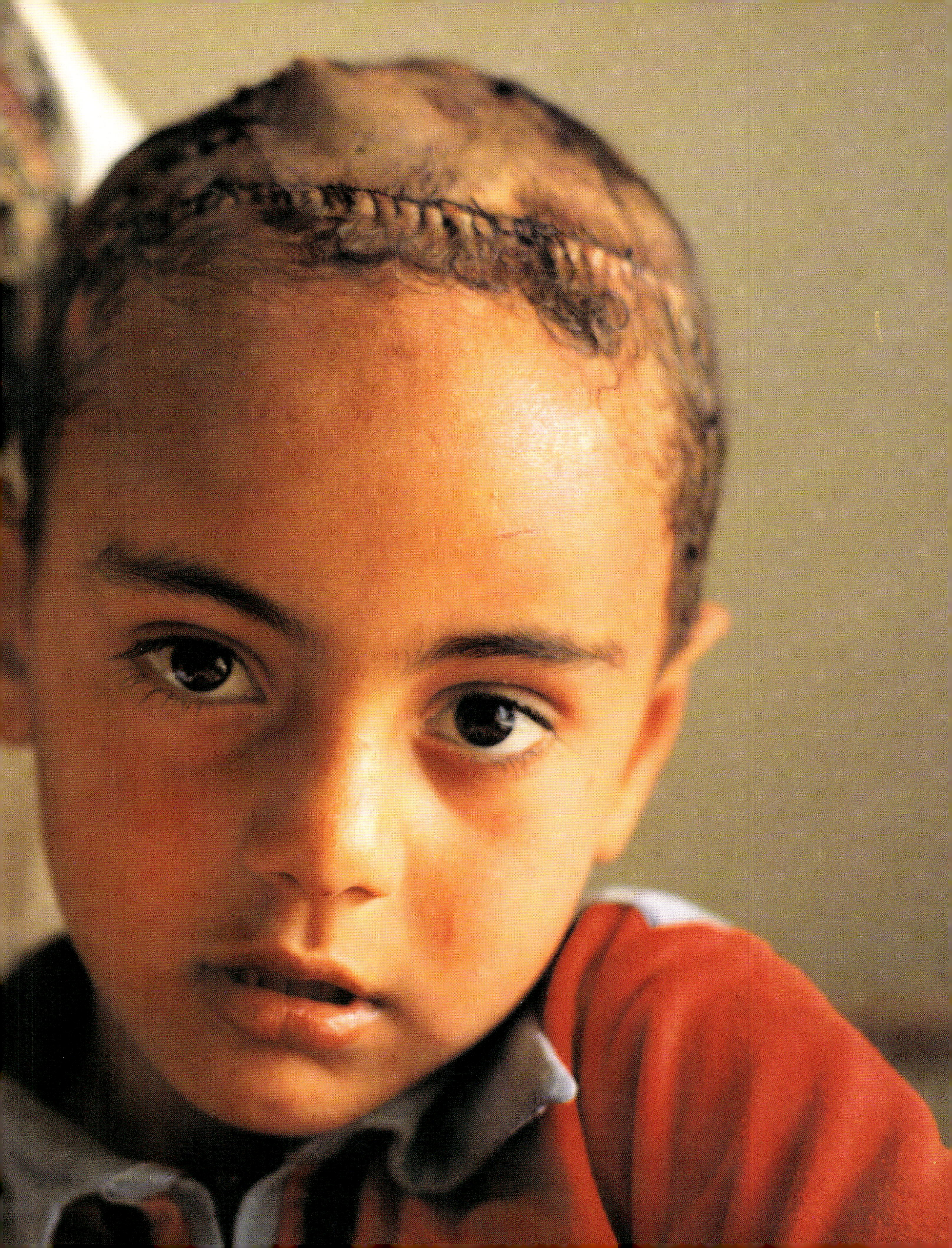

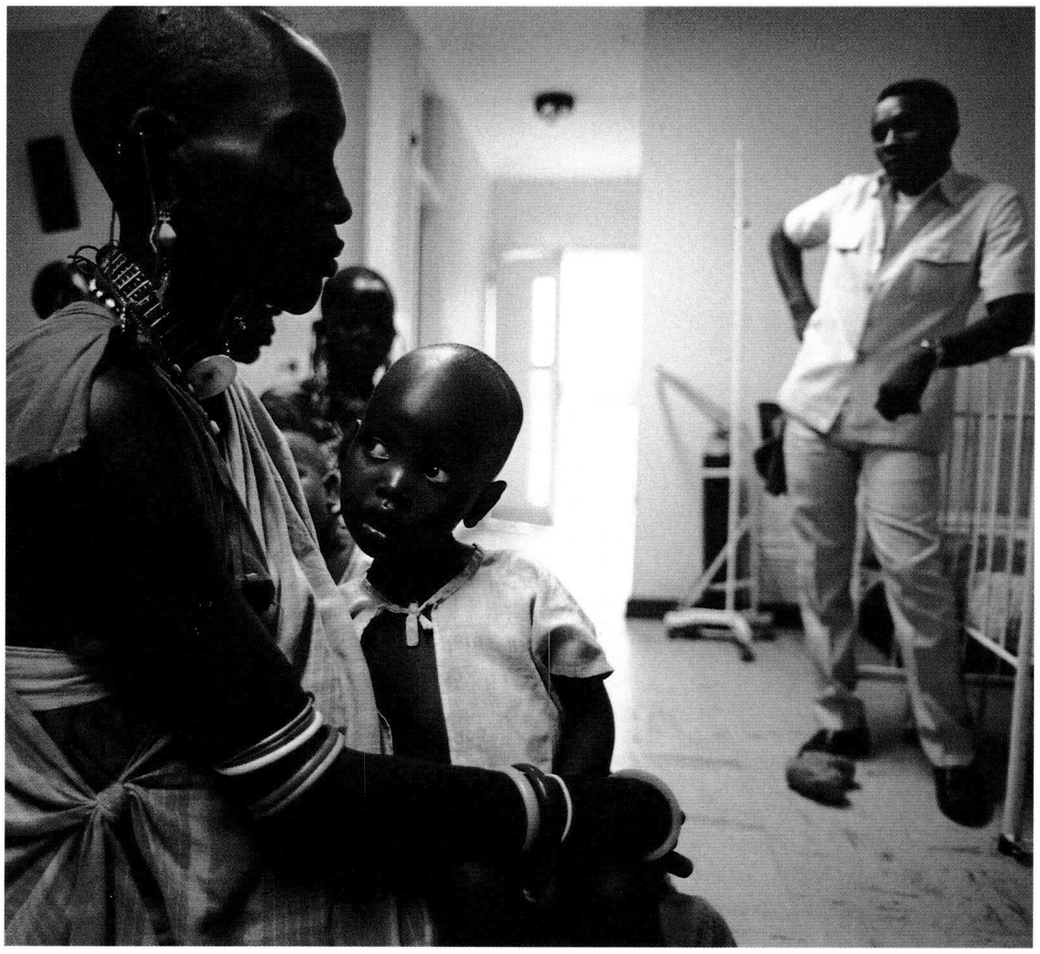

screening room, outpost hospital, Kenya
(previous spread) patient with mother, Jerusalem

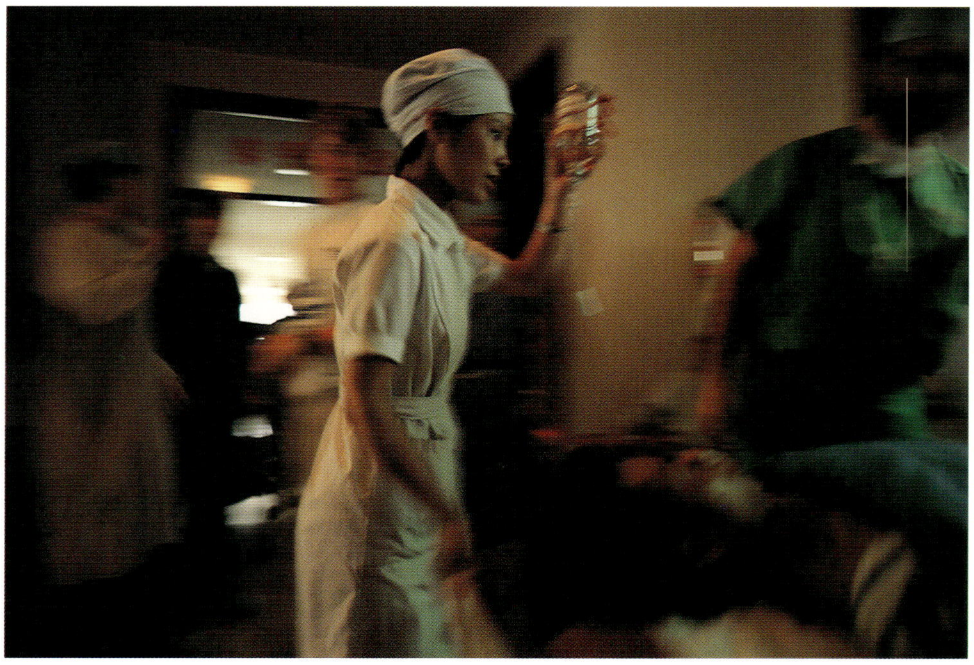

leaving recovery room, Hangzhou

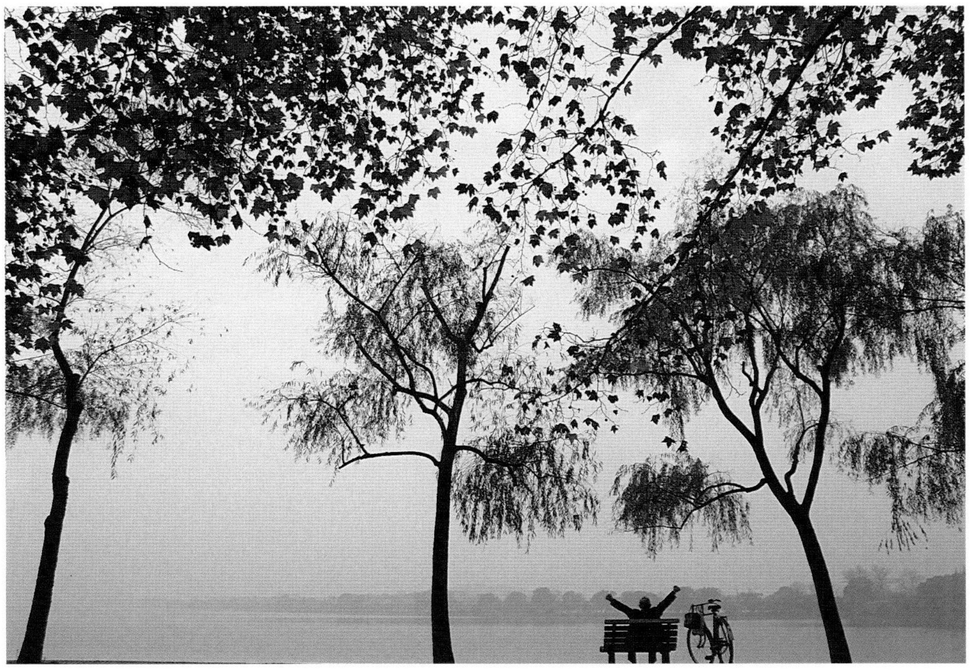

morning on West Lake, Hangzhou

Dedication to my doctors

Operation Smile!
yes, dear doctors, men of altruism,
you fly in the sky
across the Pacific ocean
to this side of sorrowful people
to give any child
who never knows the smile before
a certain smile!

Thank you
thank you so much
I am crying while I write these lines...
may God bless you

TRAN HUO LONG
FATHER OF TRAN MINH QUAN
VIETNAM

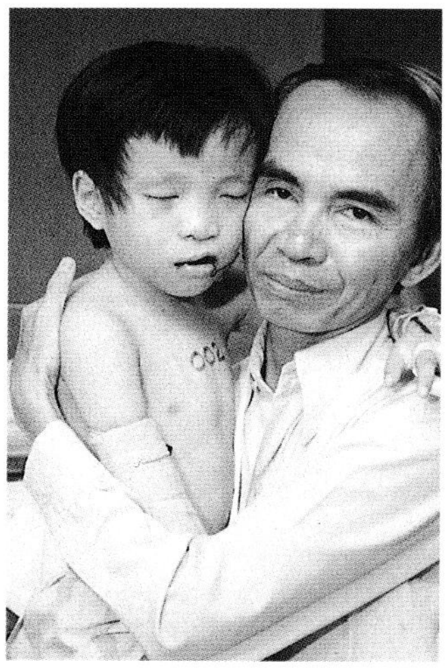

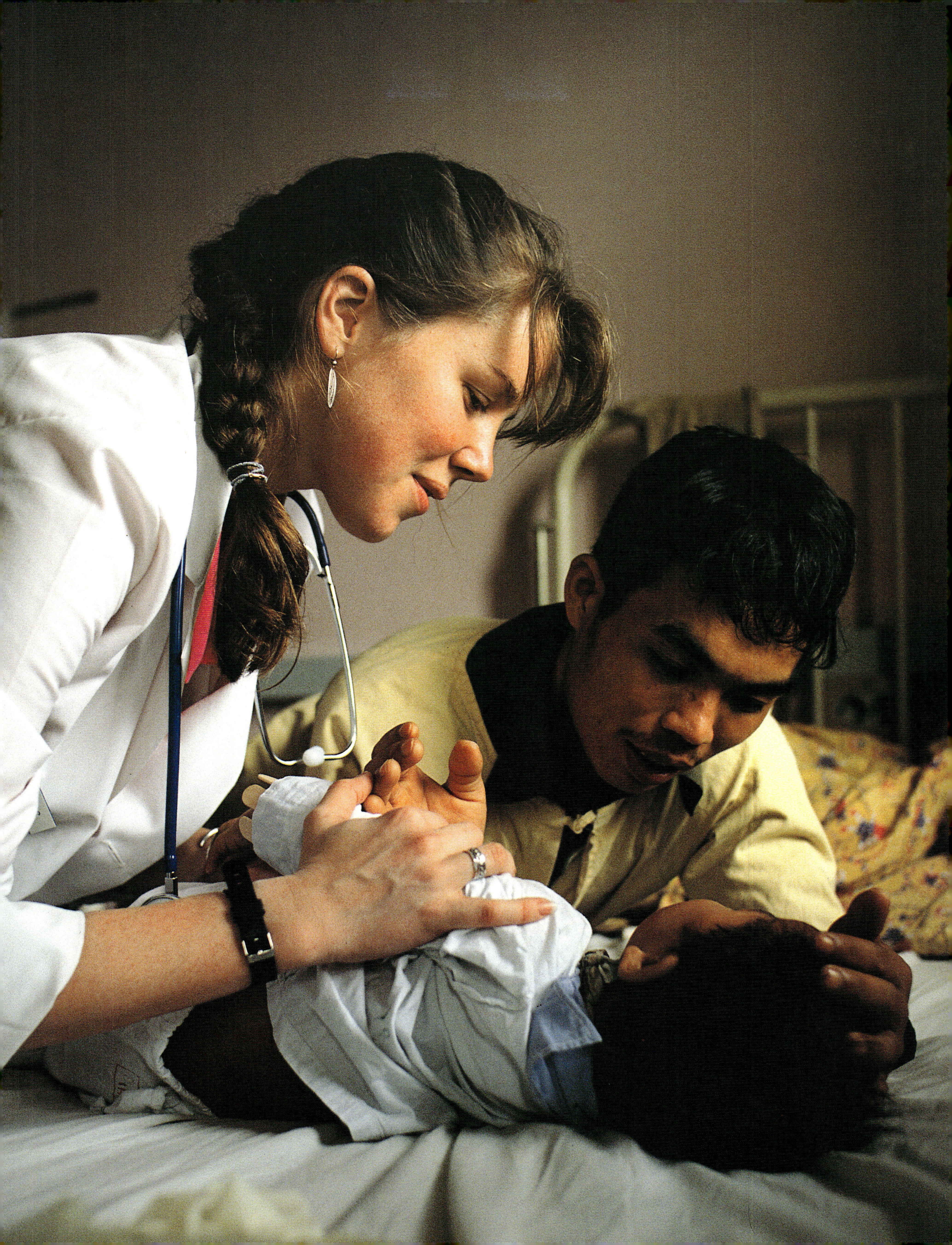

(previous page) recovery room, Hanoi

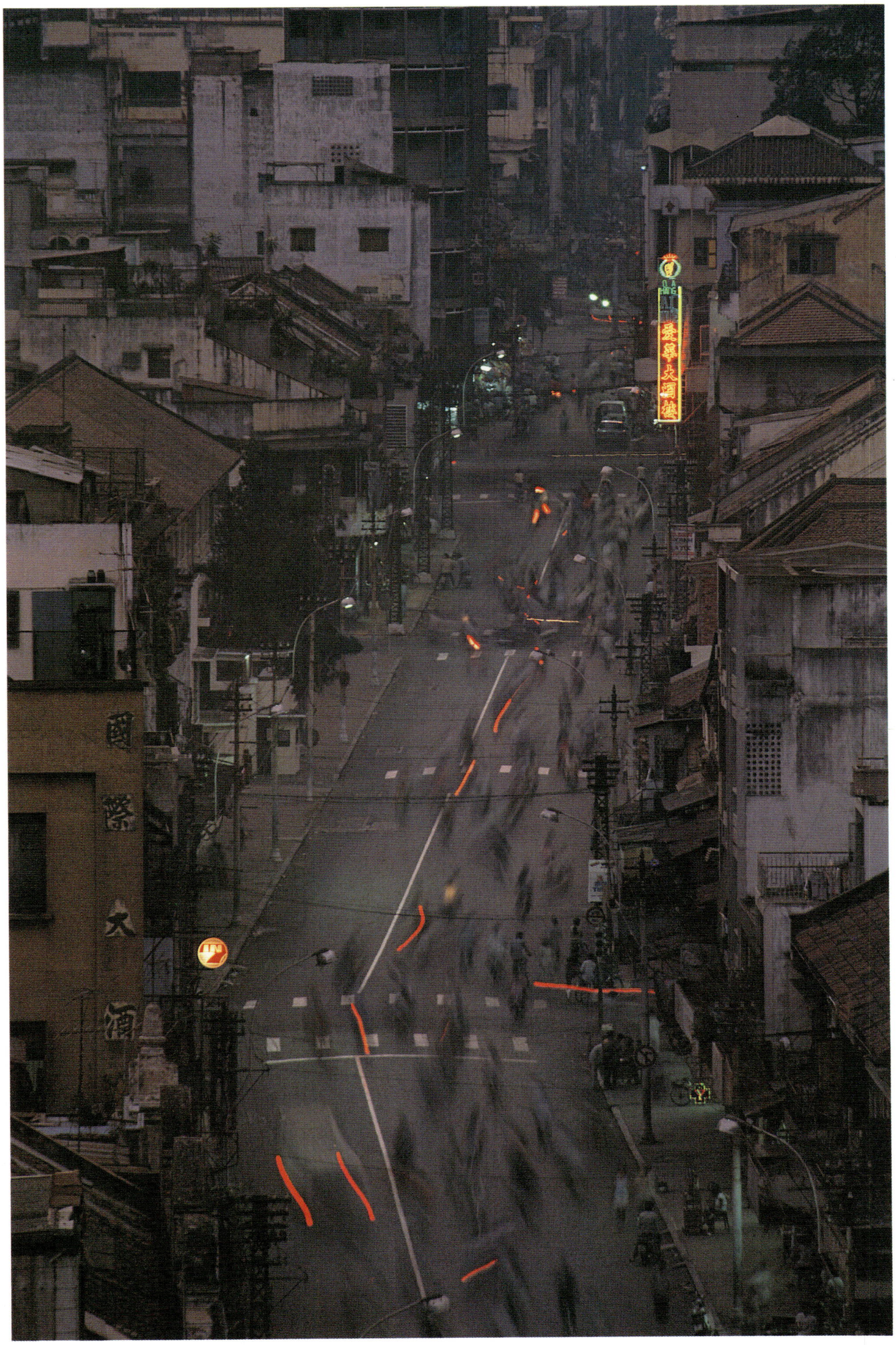

dusk in the Chinatown section, Saigon

Operation Smile has touched the lives and hearts
of so many people in my country
with your deep caring and joyful giving.

As you give back to the children
the beauty and warmth of their smiles,
our people, edified by your generosity,
look now to the future when they can join you
as partners in your missions of love.

PRESIDENT CORAZON C. AQUINO
REPUBLIC OF THE PHILIPPINES

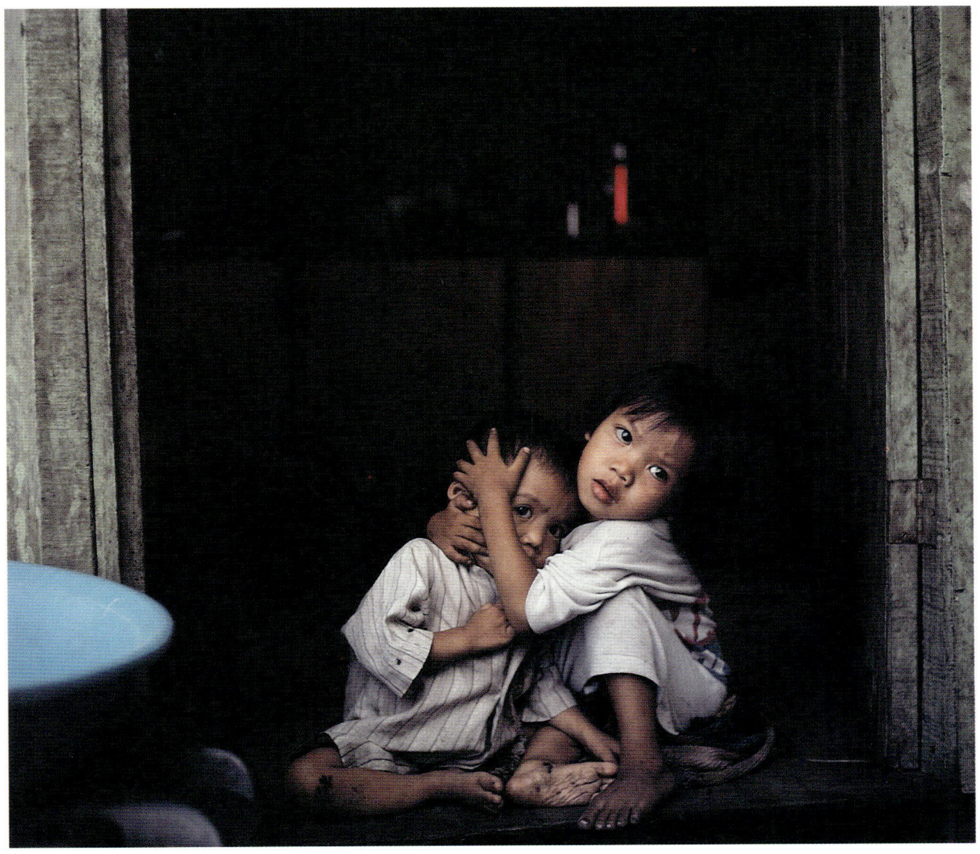

children, metro Manila dump

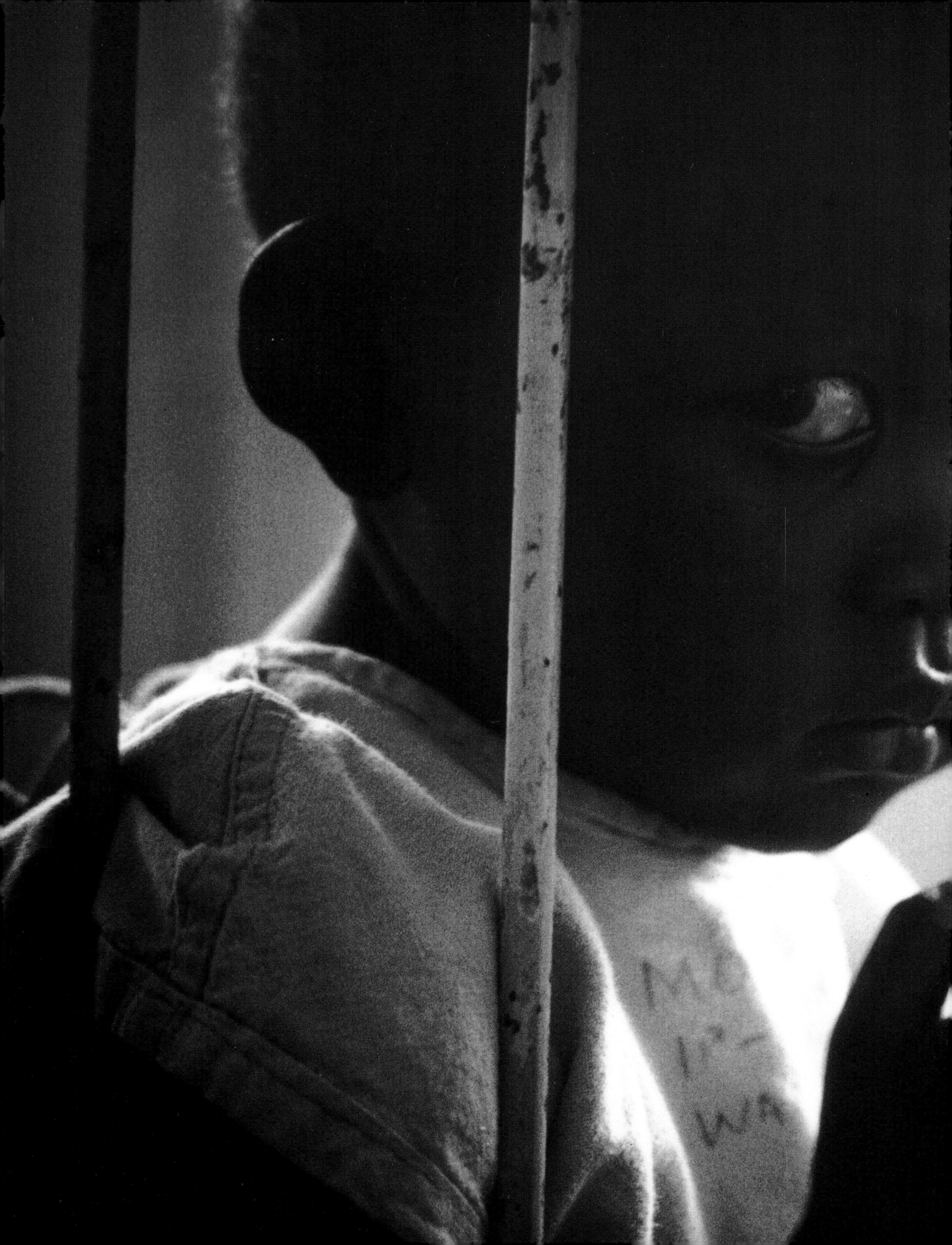

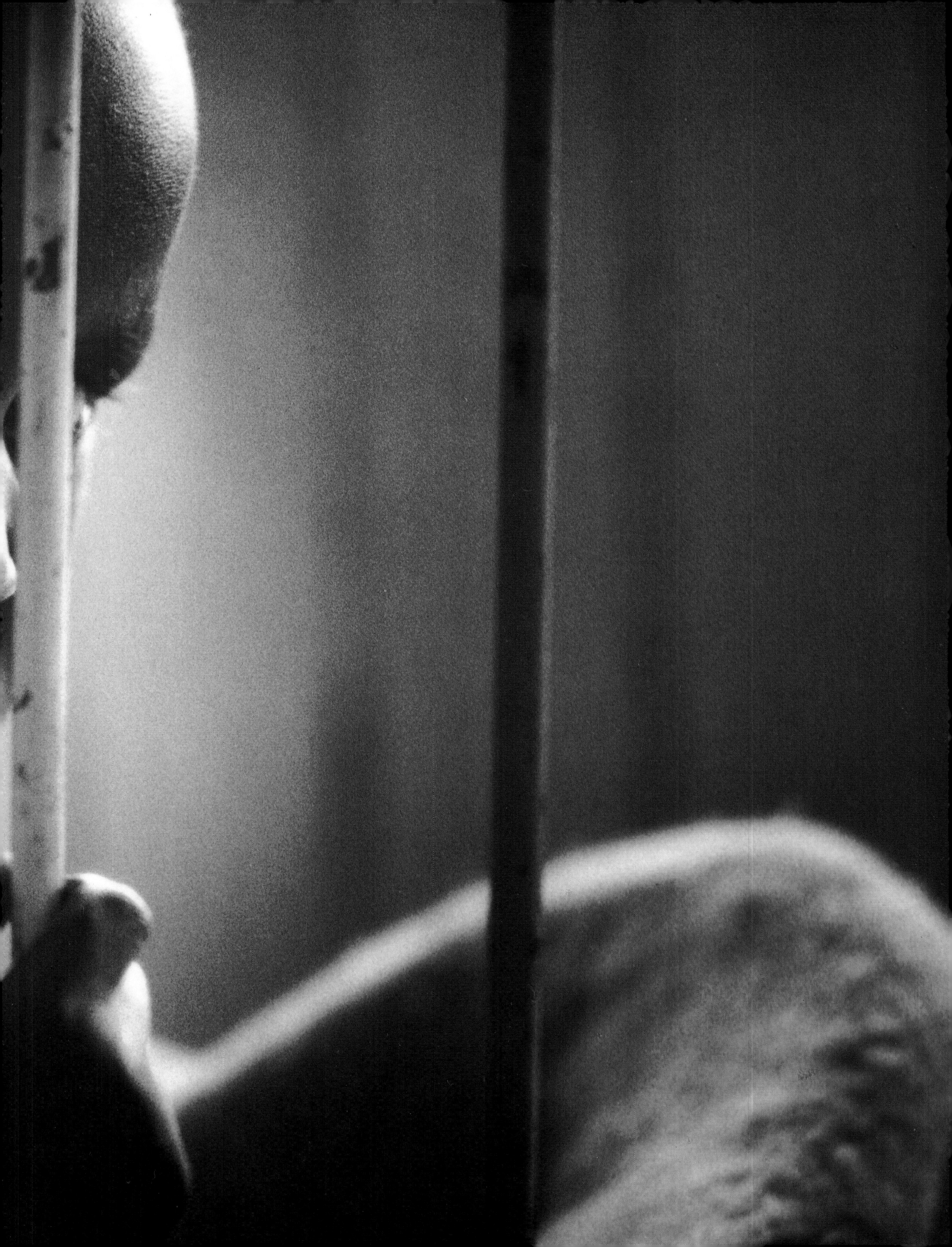

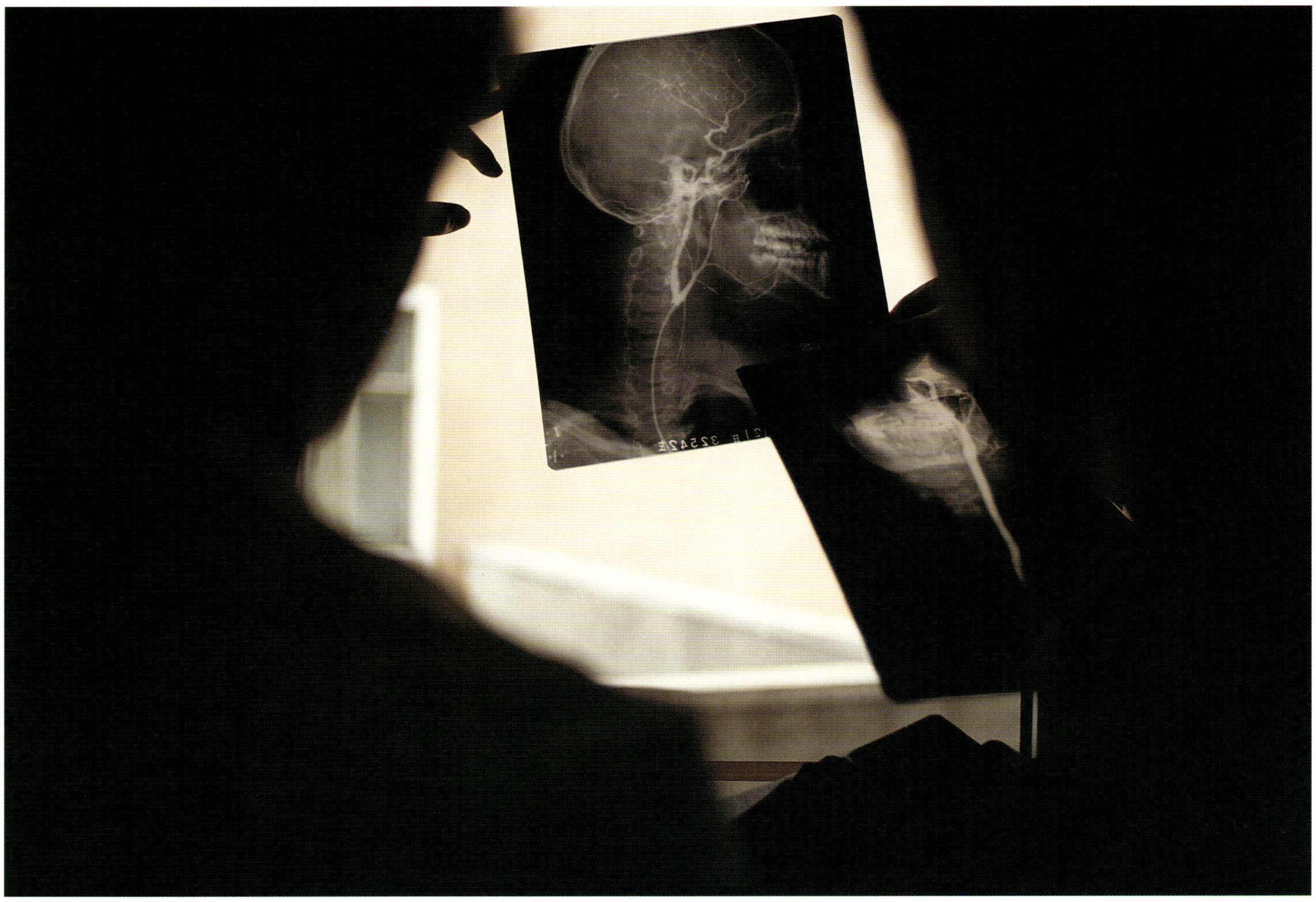

Xrays, Hangzhou
(previous spread) boy in crib, Nairobi

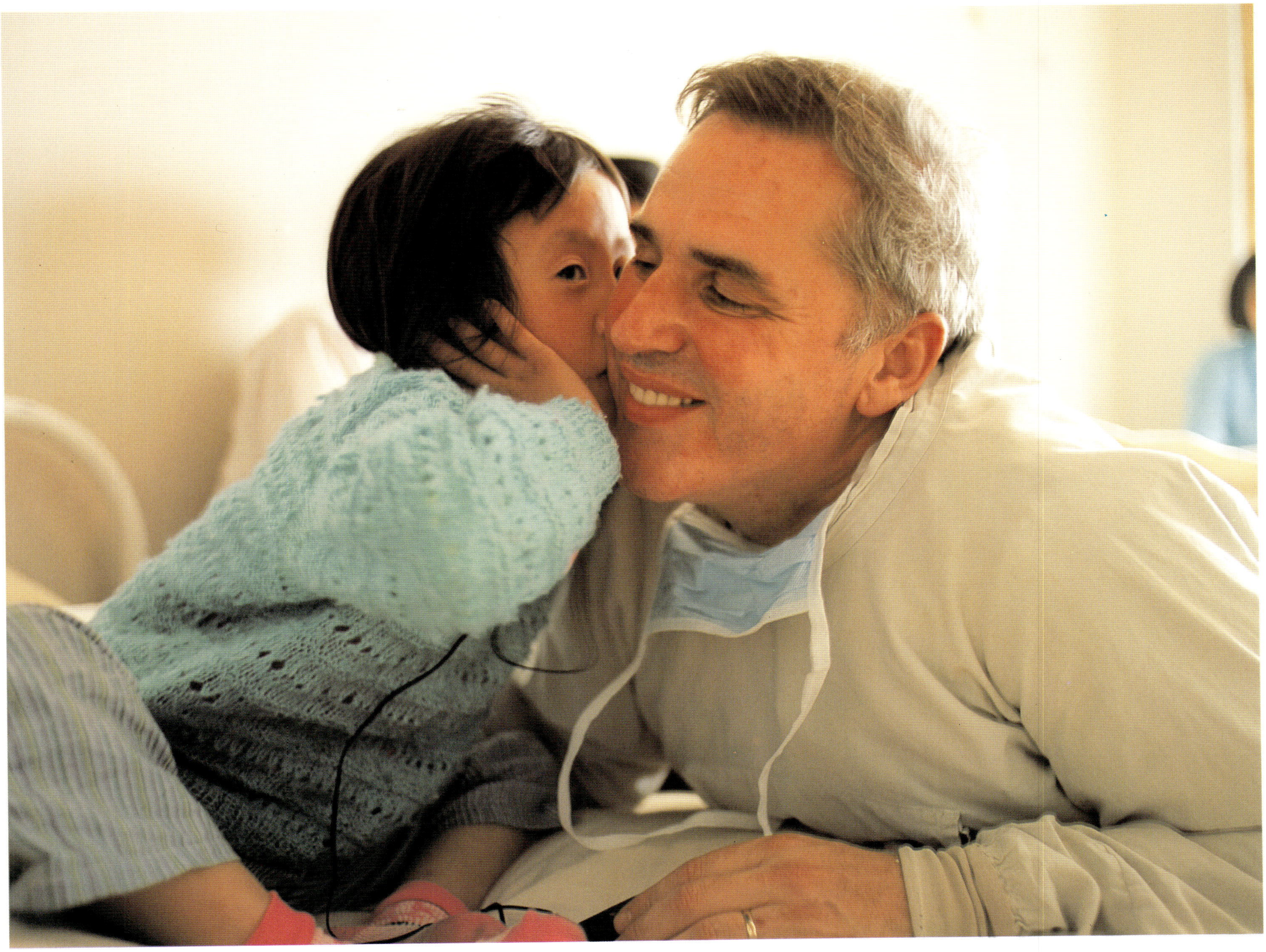

post-op ward, Hangzhou

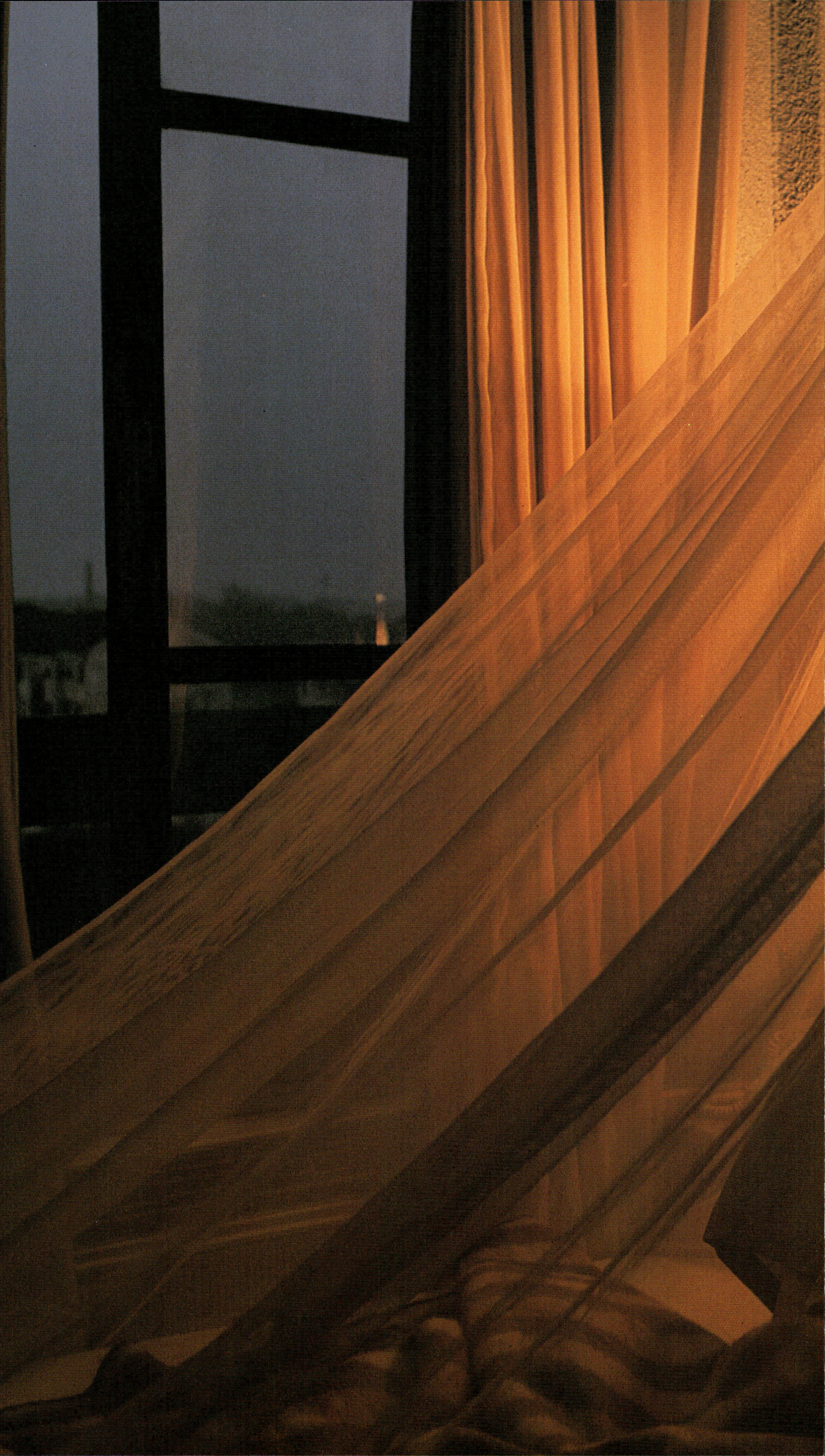

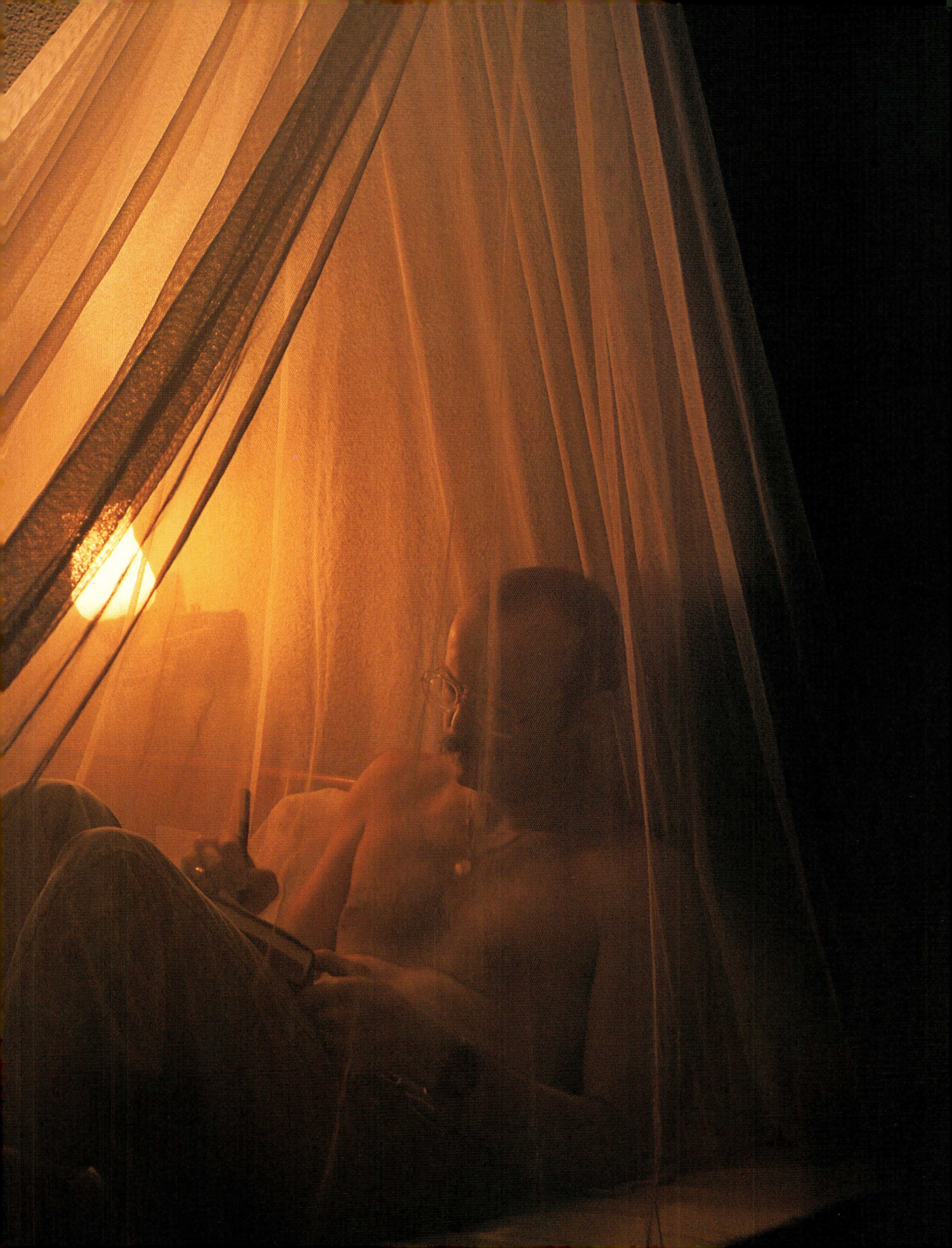

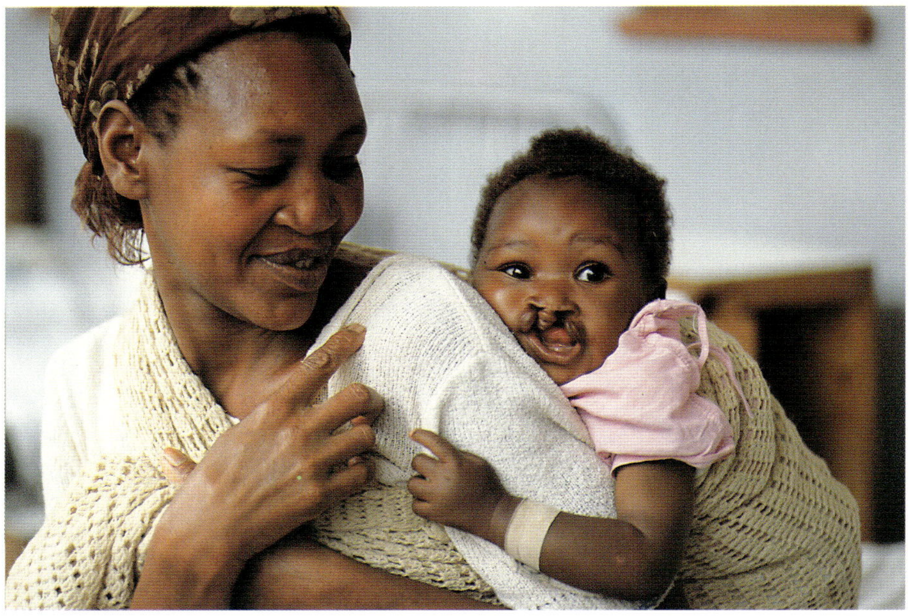

patient with mother, Nairobi
photograph by Barbara Kinney
(previous spread) volunteer doctor, before sunrise, Hanoi

Despite monstrous facial distortion,
their wide-eyed innocence staring up at us
revealed an inner beauty shared only by children.

MORTON H. GOLDSTEIN, MD
OSI MEDICAL VOLUNTEER

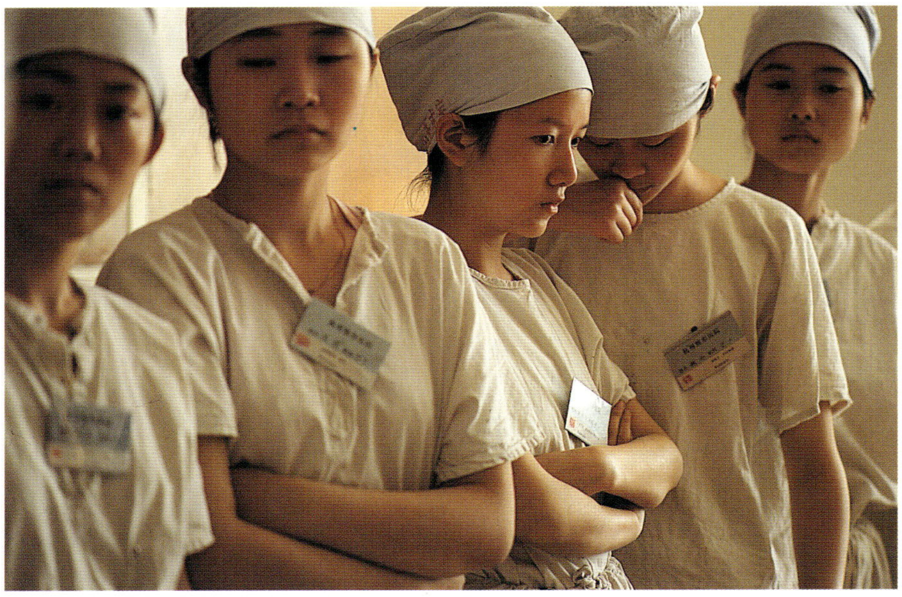

nurses receiving orders, Hangzhou

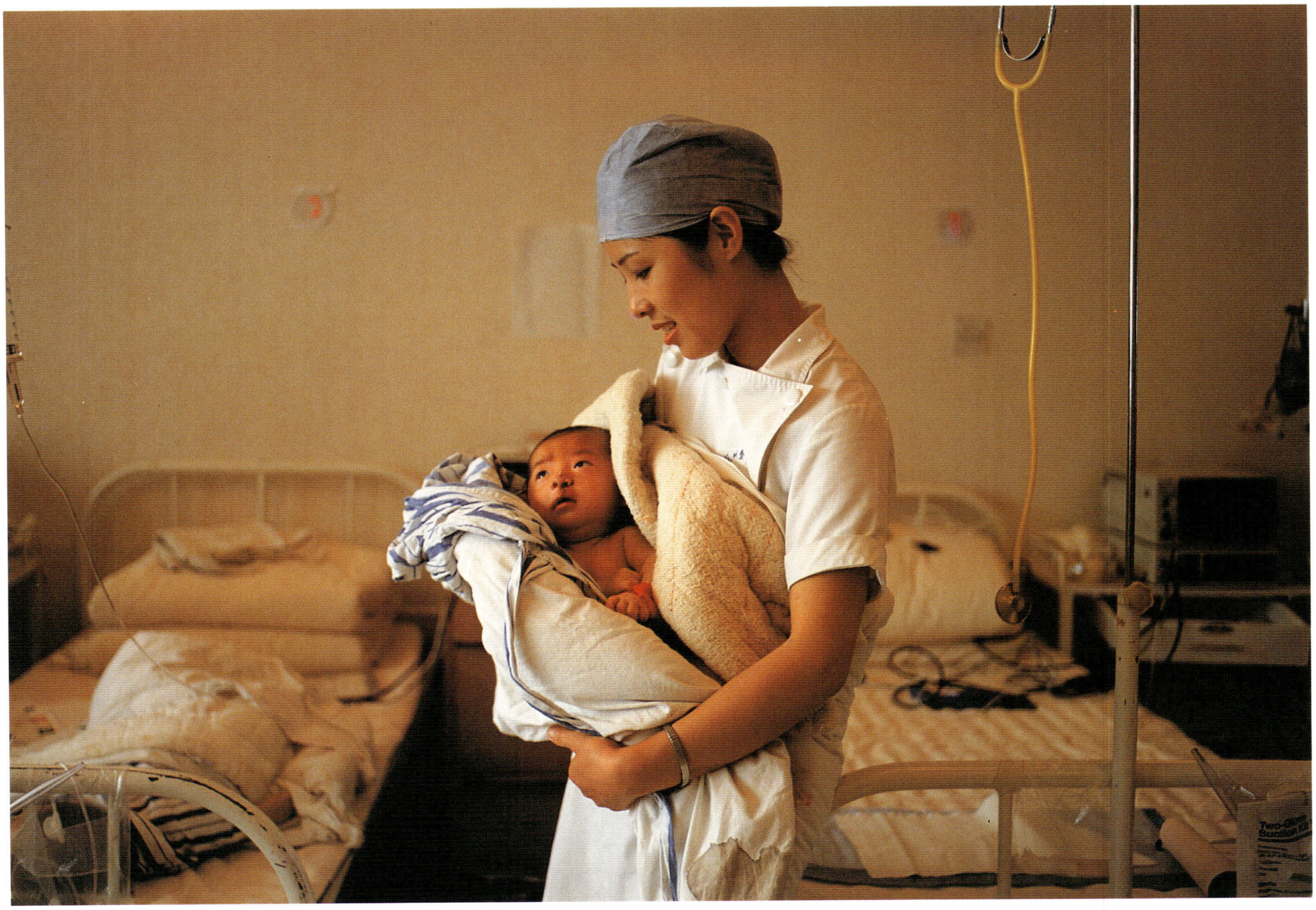

recovery room, Hangzhou

boy on the roadside, Monrovia

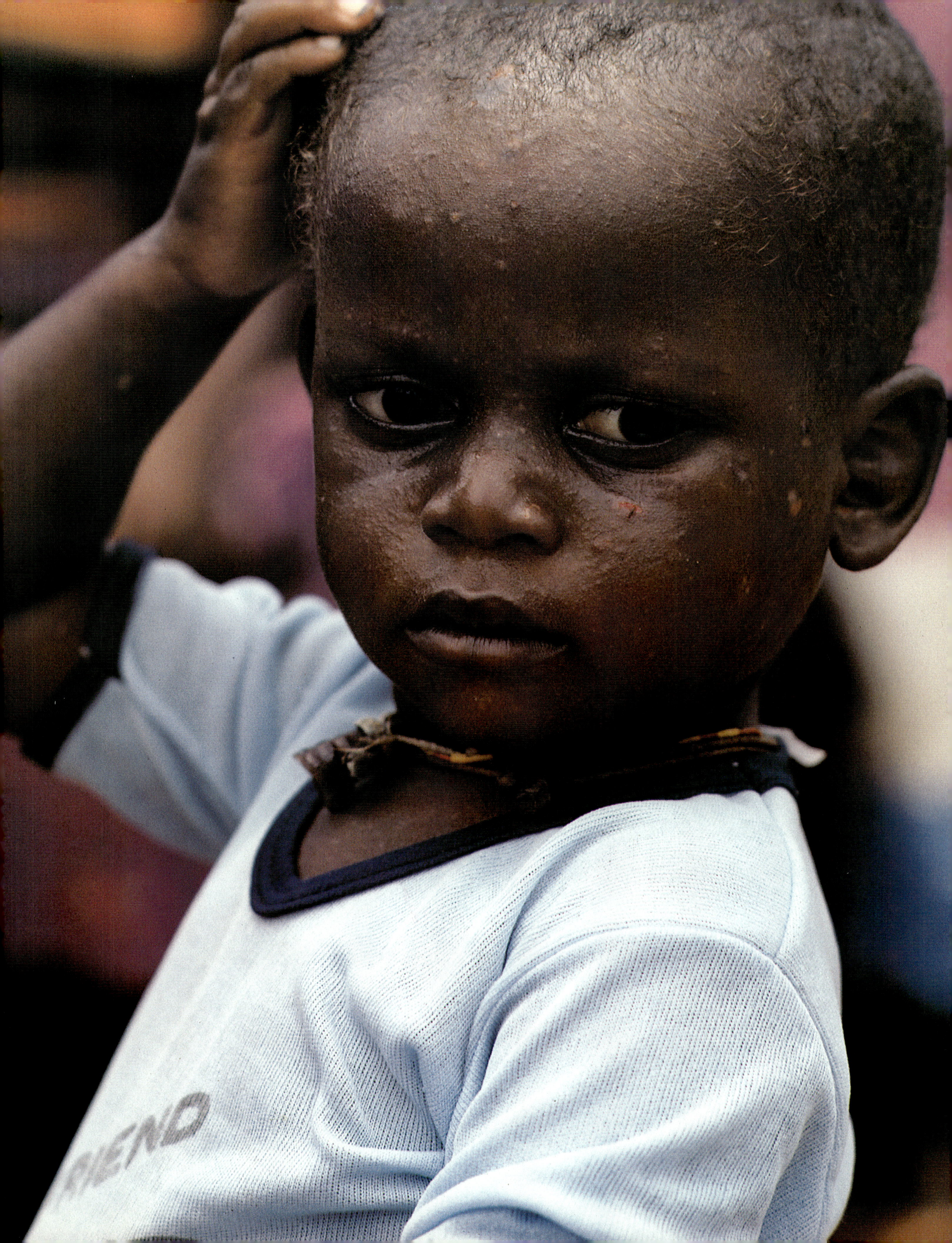

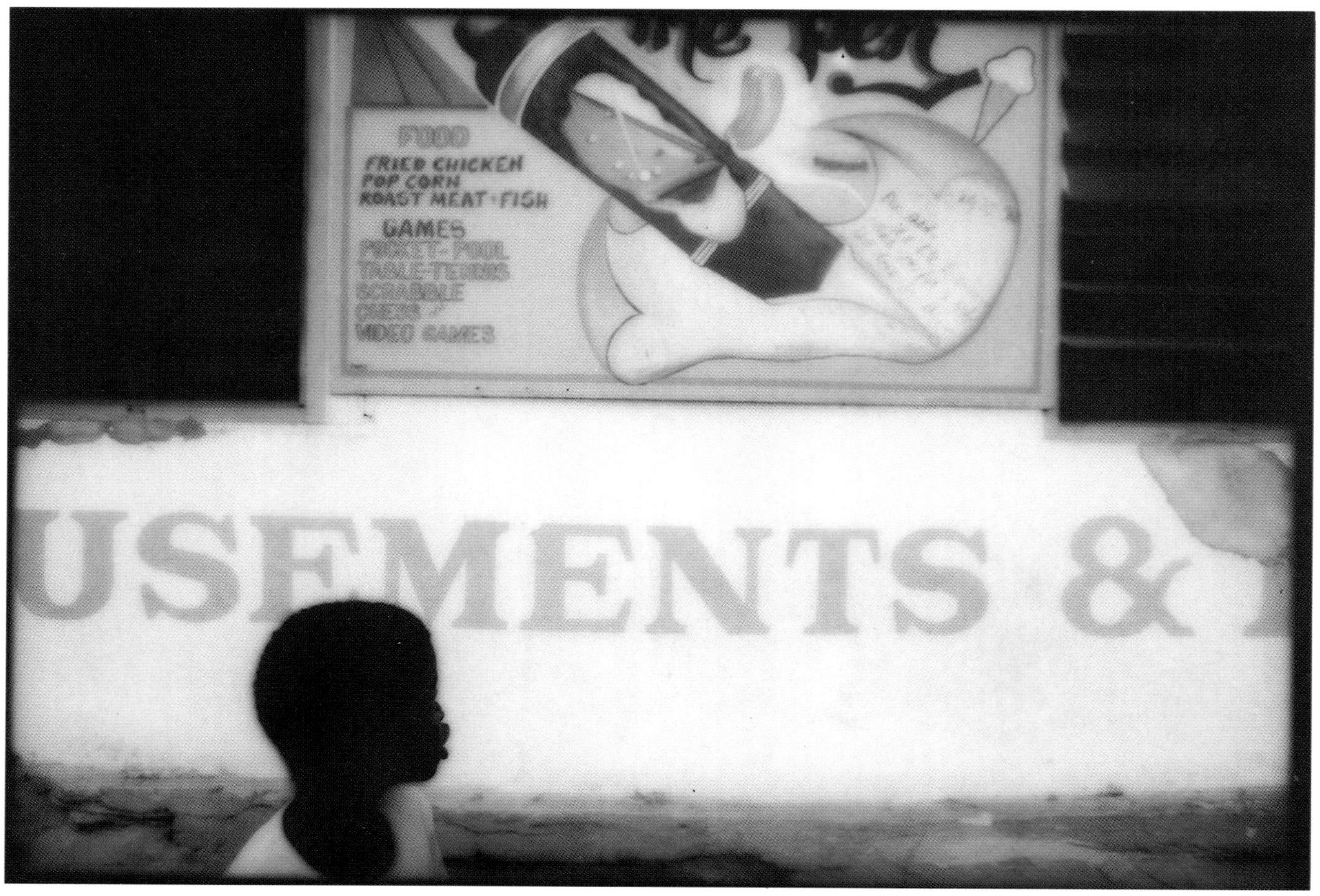
FOOD
FRIED CHICKEN
POP CORN
ROAST MEAT · FISH
GAMES
POCKET-POOL
TABLE-TENNIS
SCRABBLE
CHESS
VIDEO GAMES
USEMENTS &

boy on the street, Monrovia

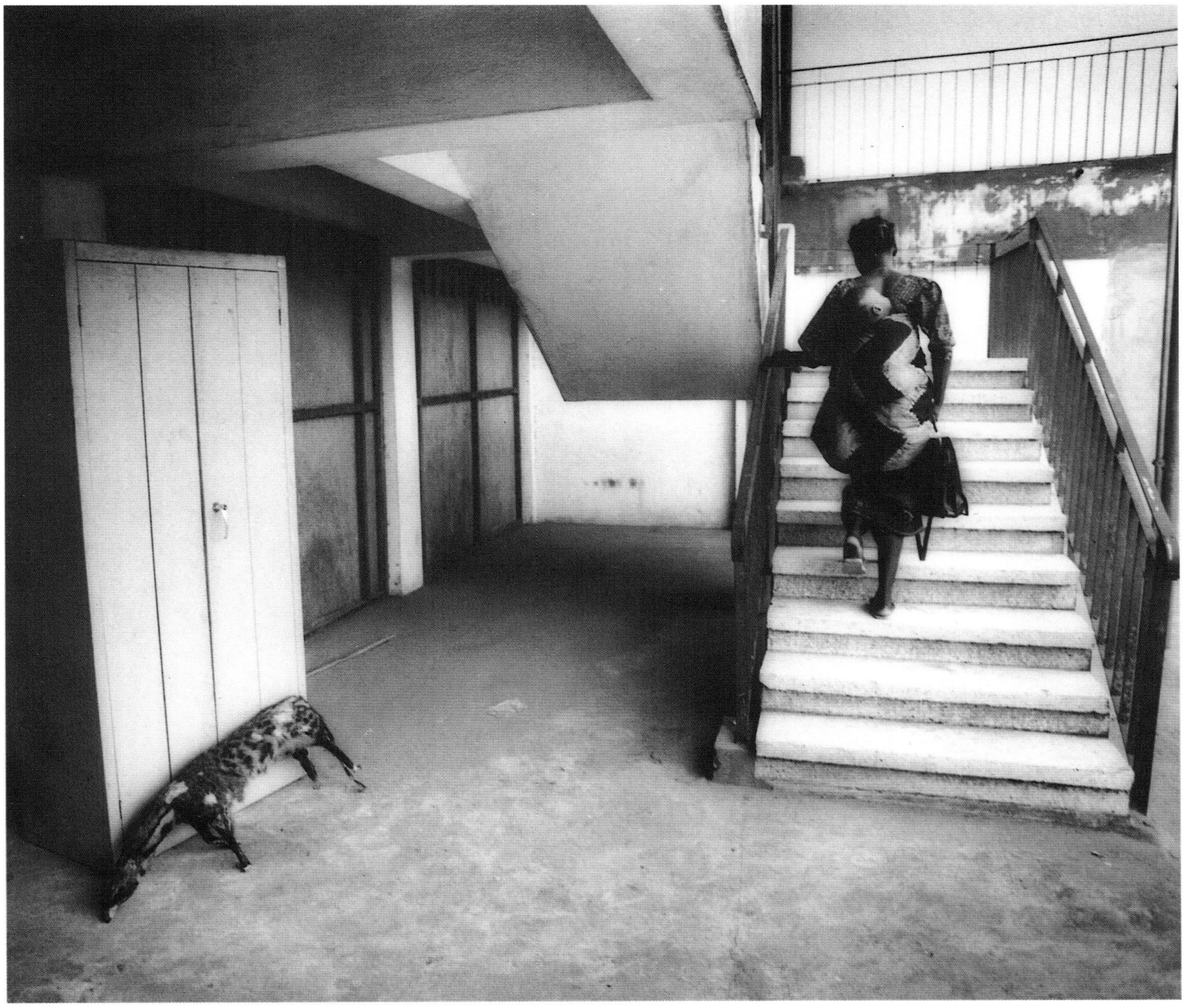

dead anteater, mother and child, Monrovia

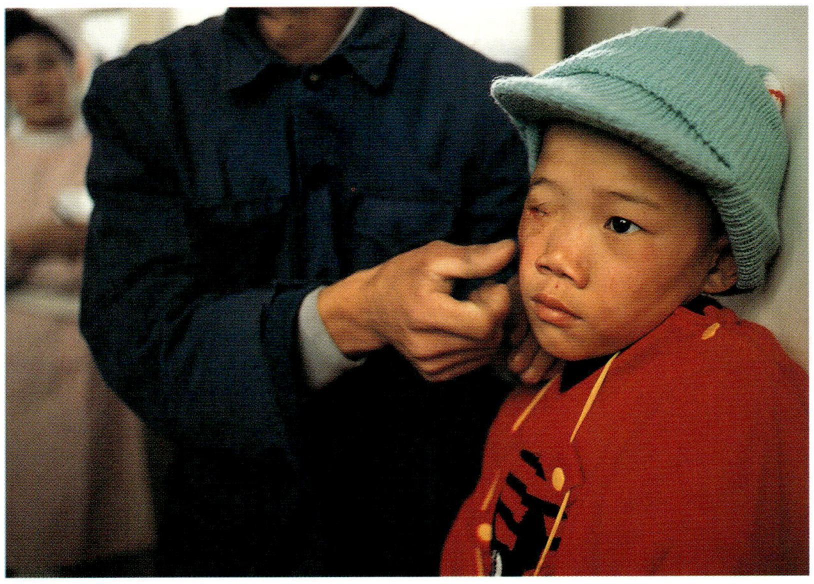

patient in screening, Hangzhou

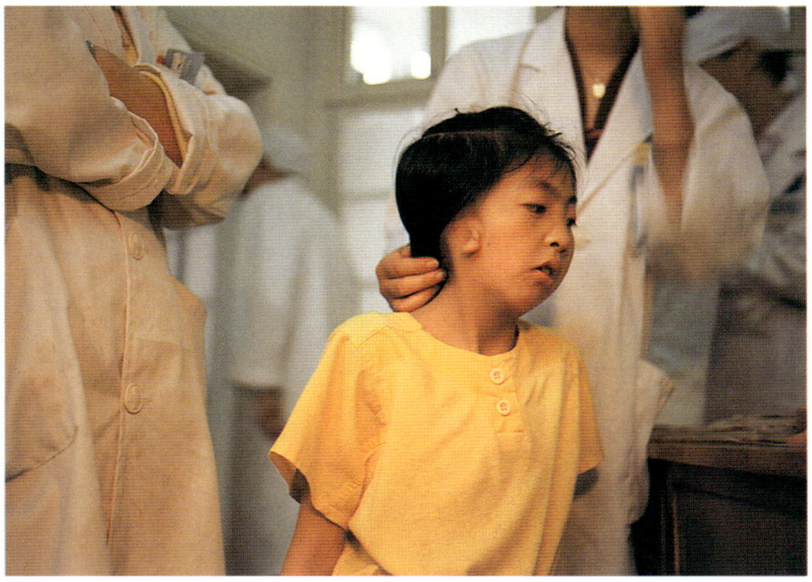

patient in screening, Hangzhou

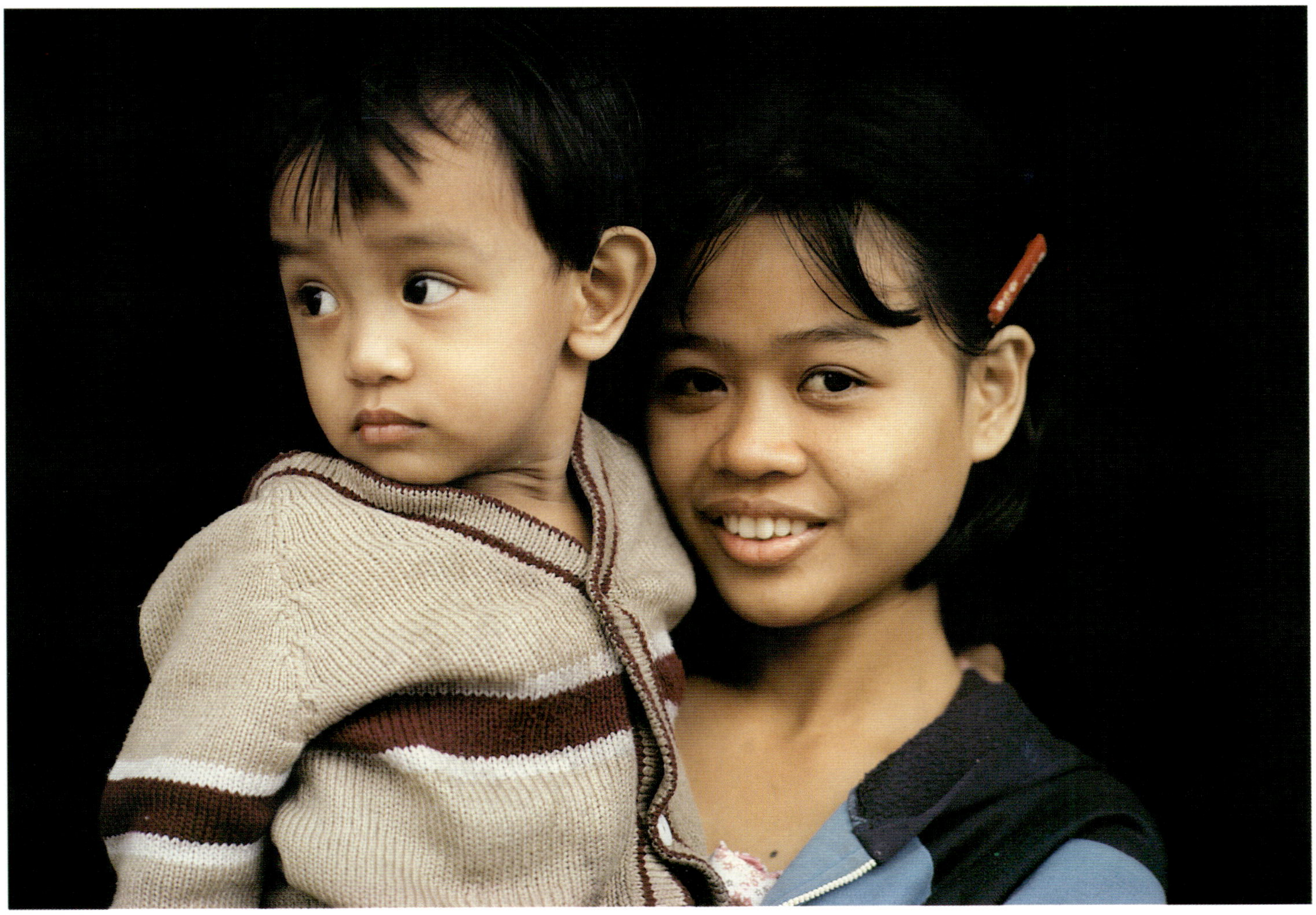

mother and child, Naga City

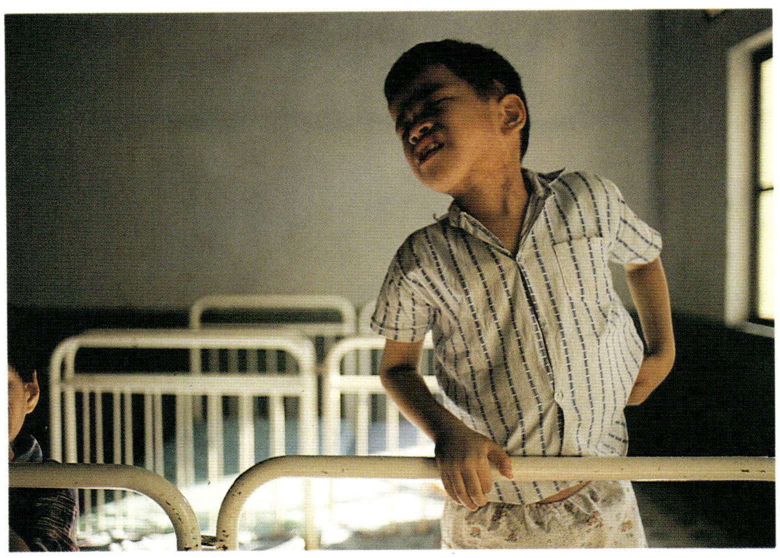

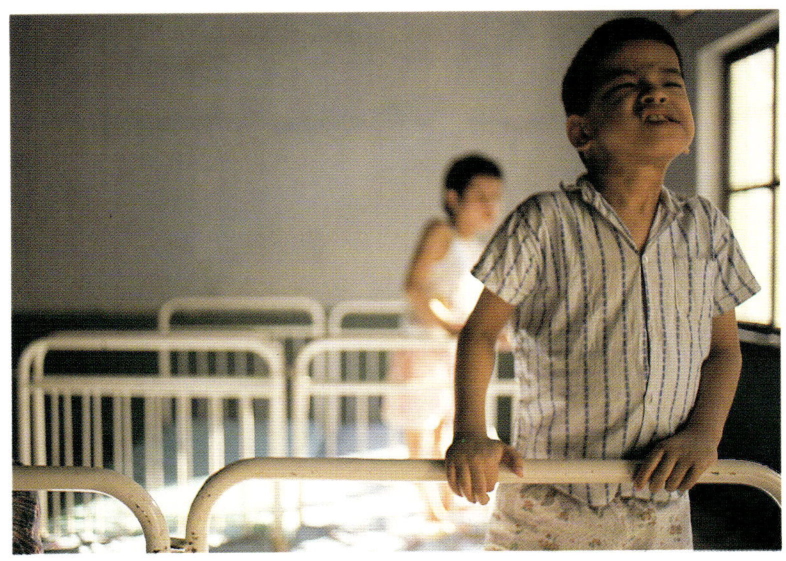

orphan at the home for retarded children, Saigon

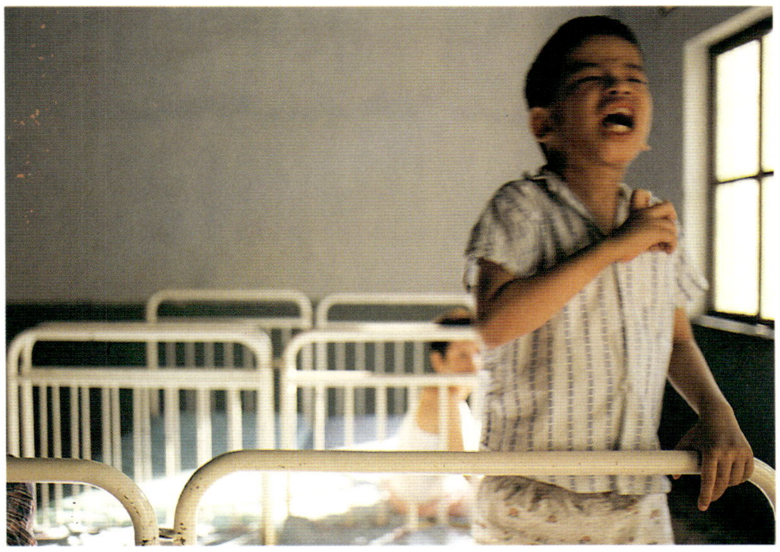 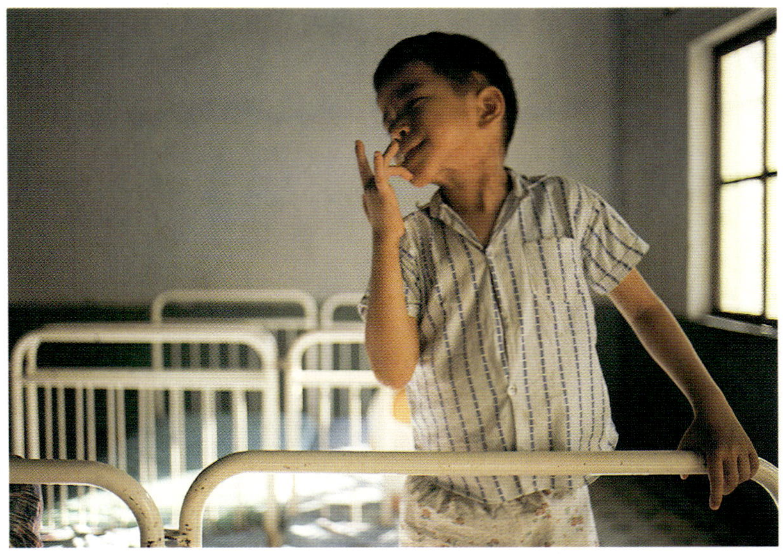

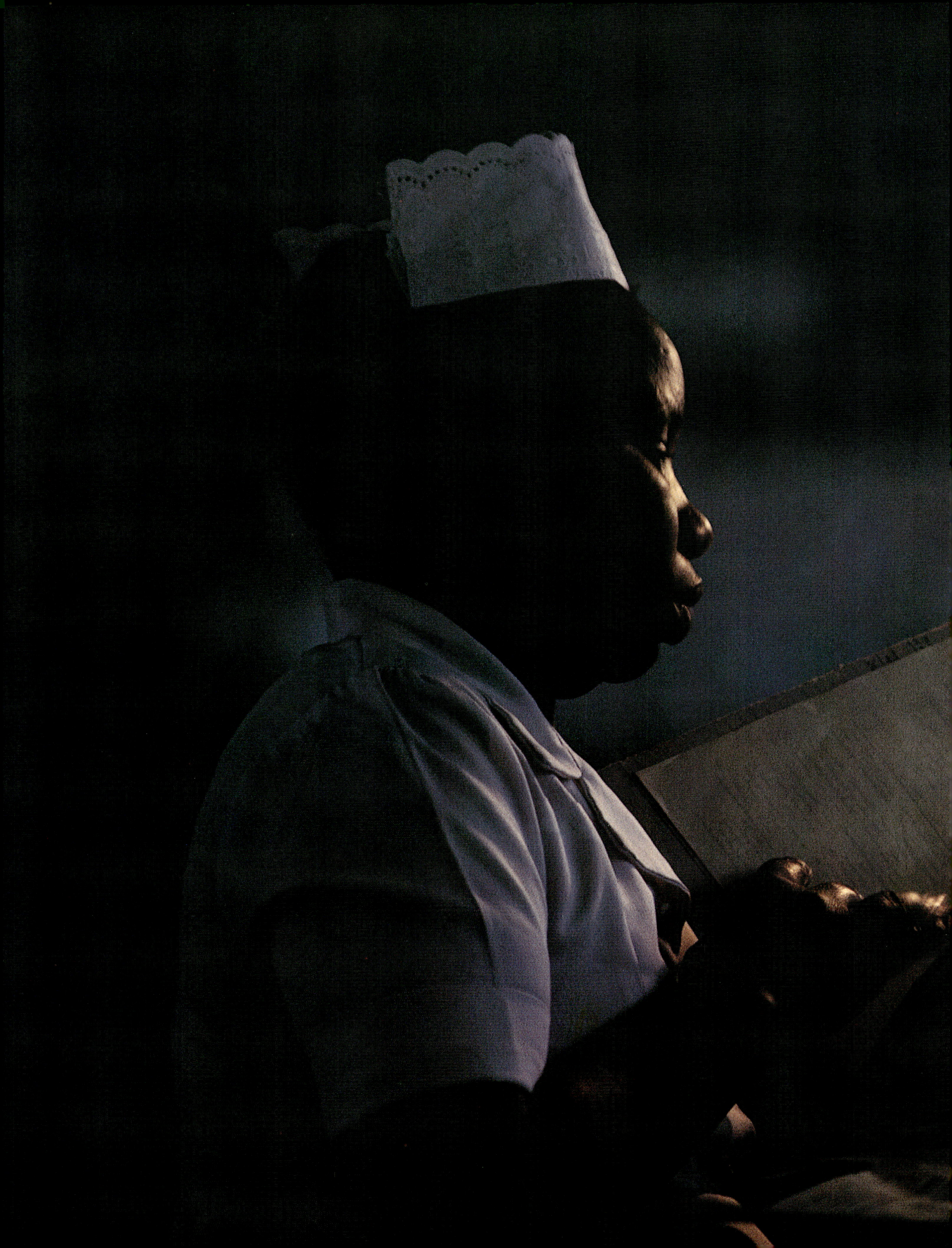

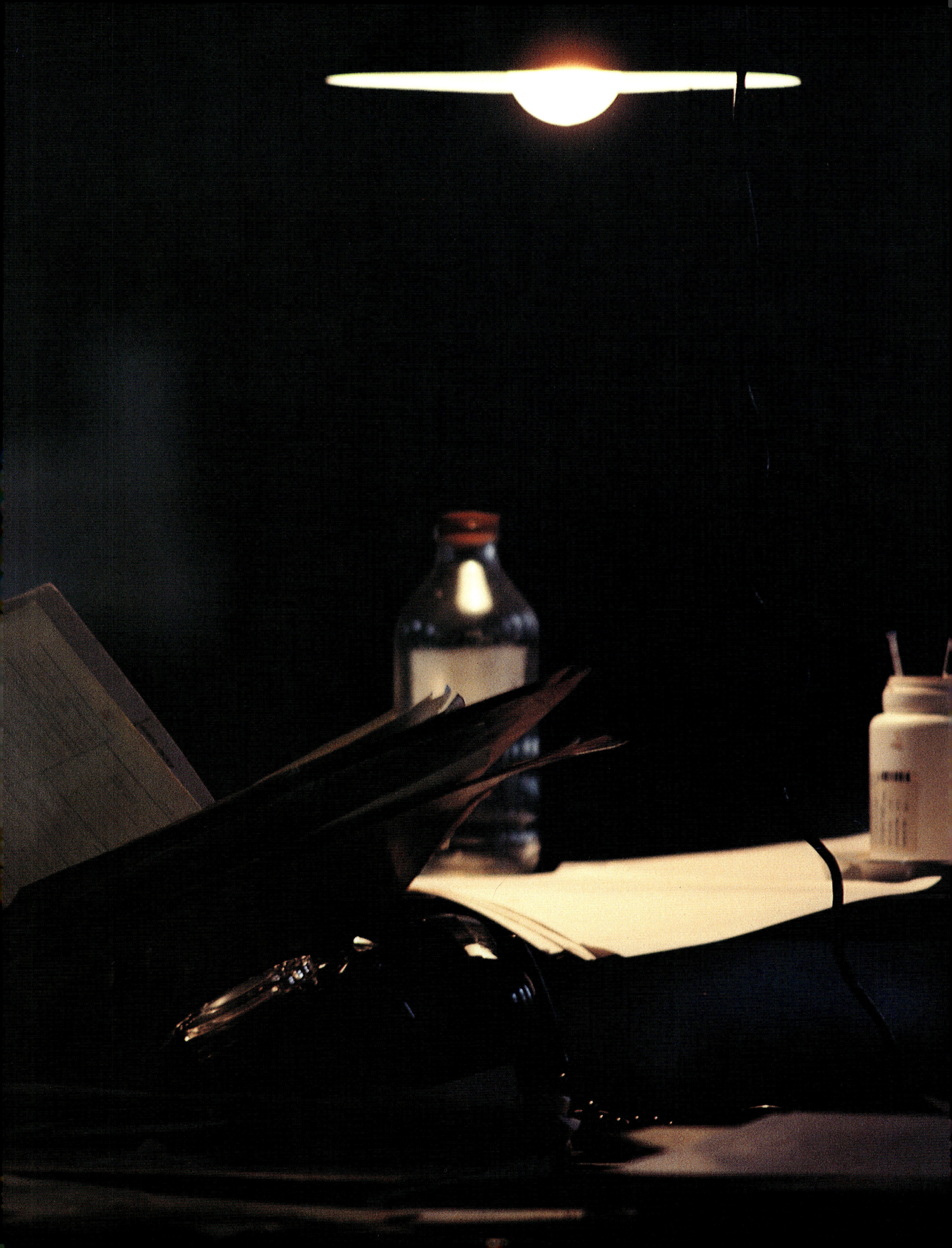

(previous spread) nurses station in pre-op ward, Nairobi

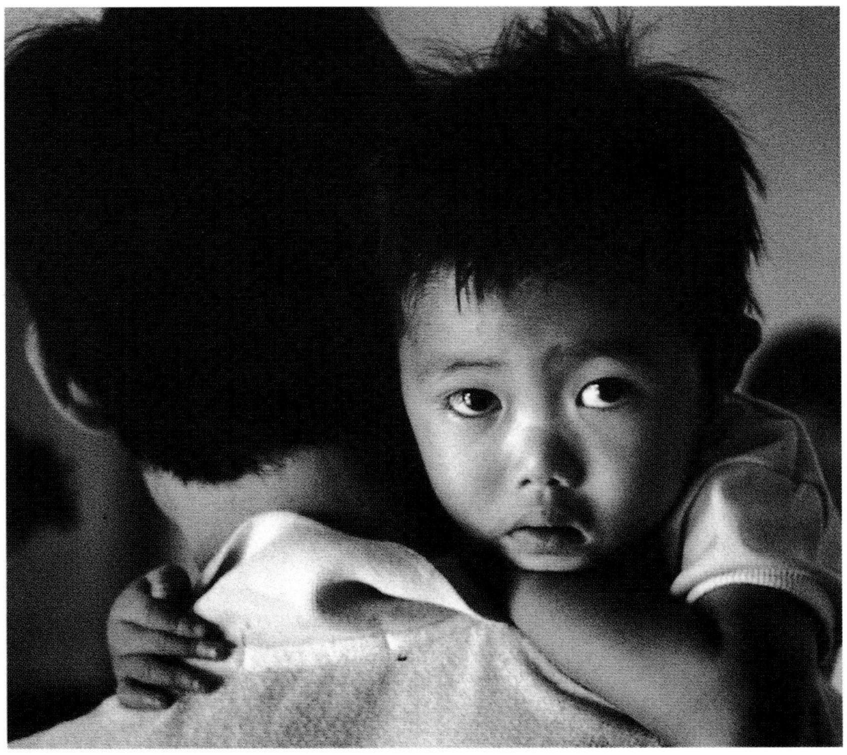

It is through the eyes of a child
that you understand the importance
of building peace in the world.

ALAIN DICK
OSI VOLUNTEER

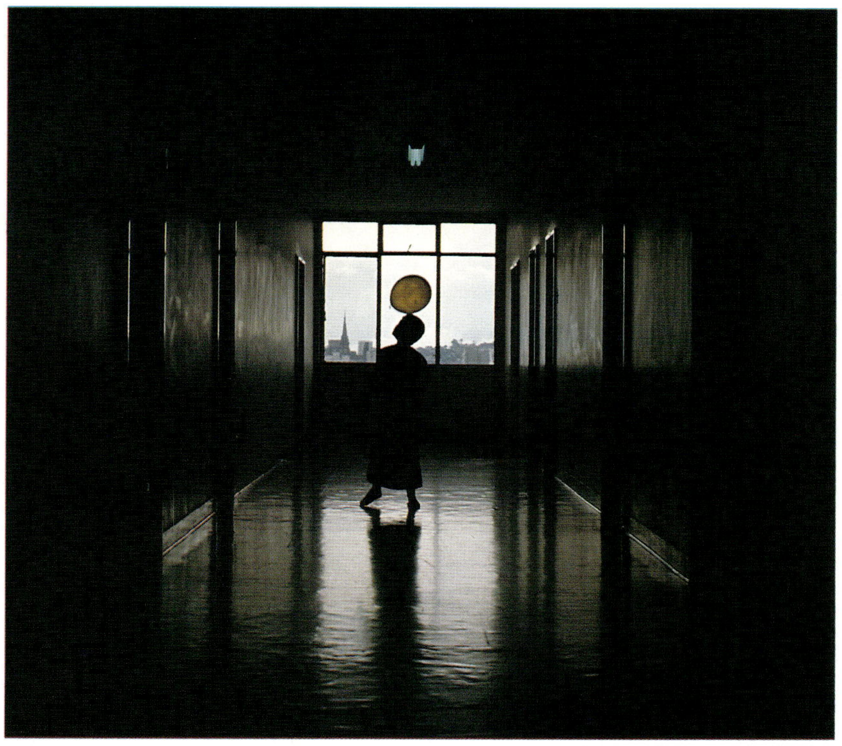

boy and balloon, children's ward, Manizales

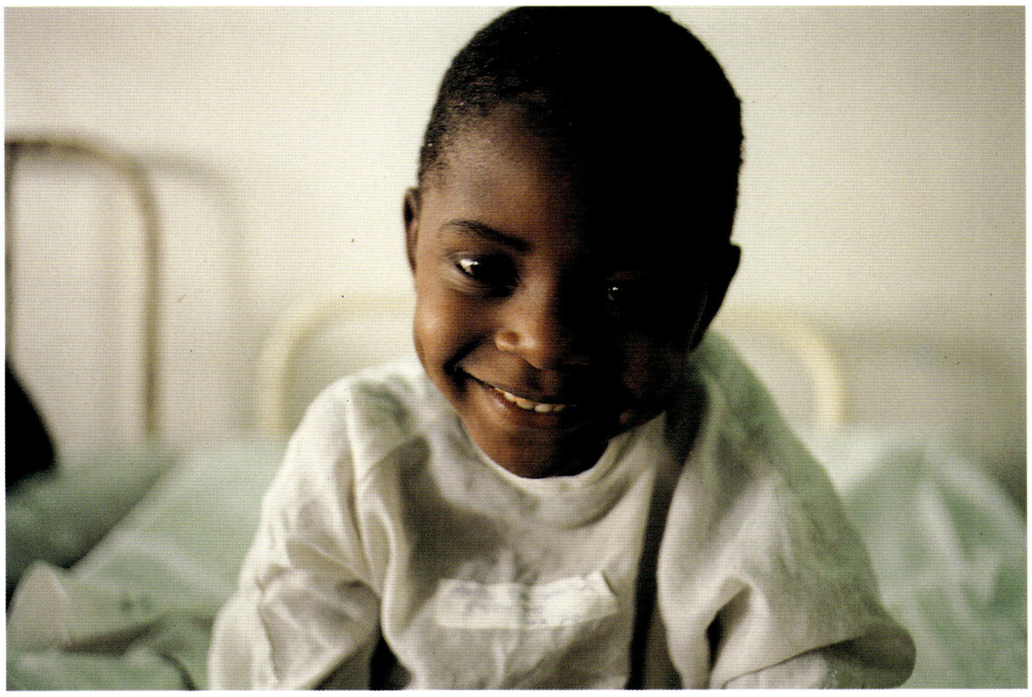

patient, Nairobi

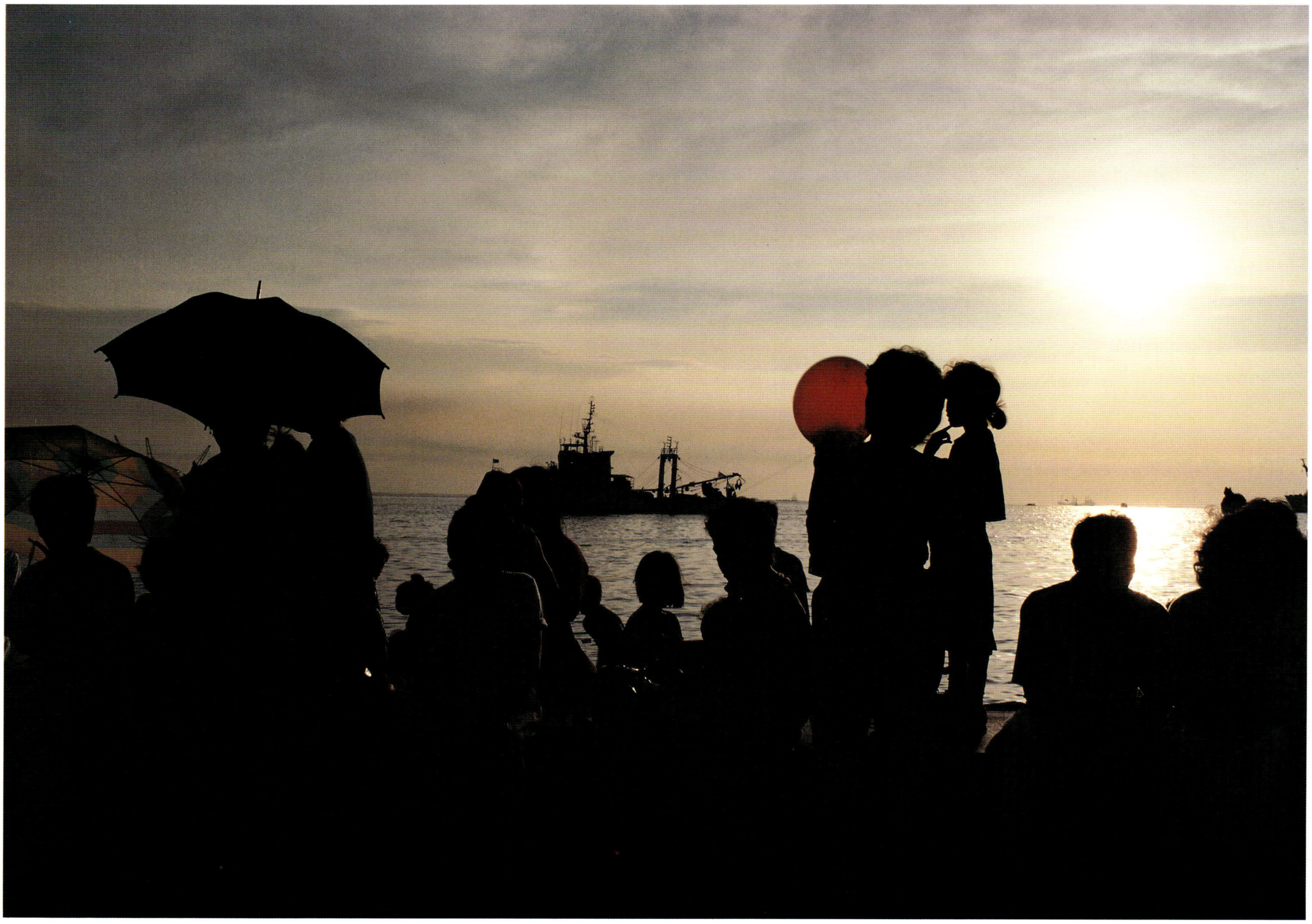

families at sunset, Manila Bay

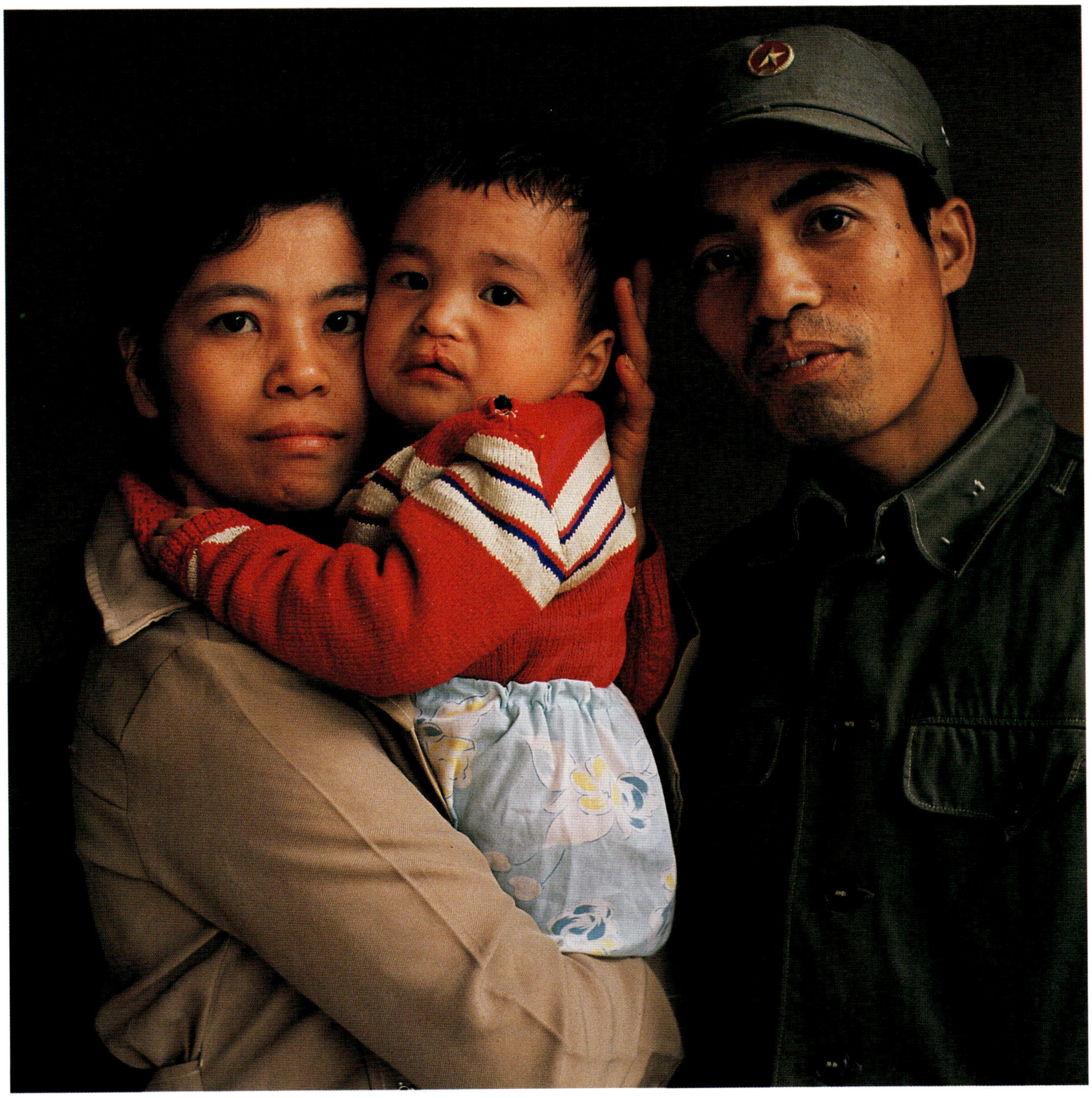

patient and parents, Hanoi

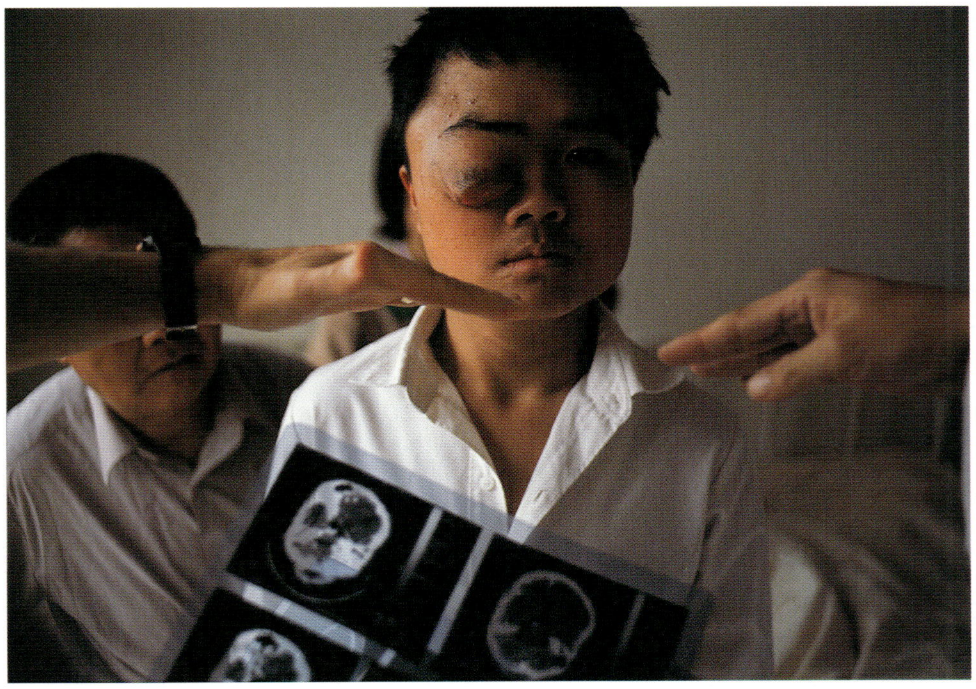

patient with X-rays, Hangzhou

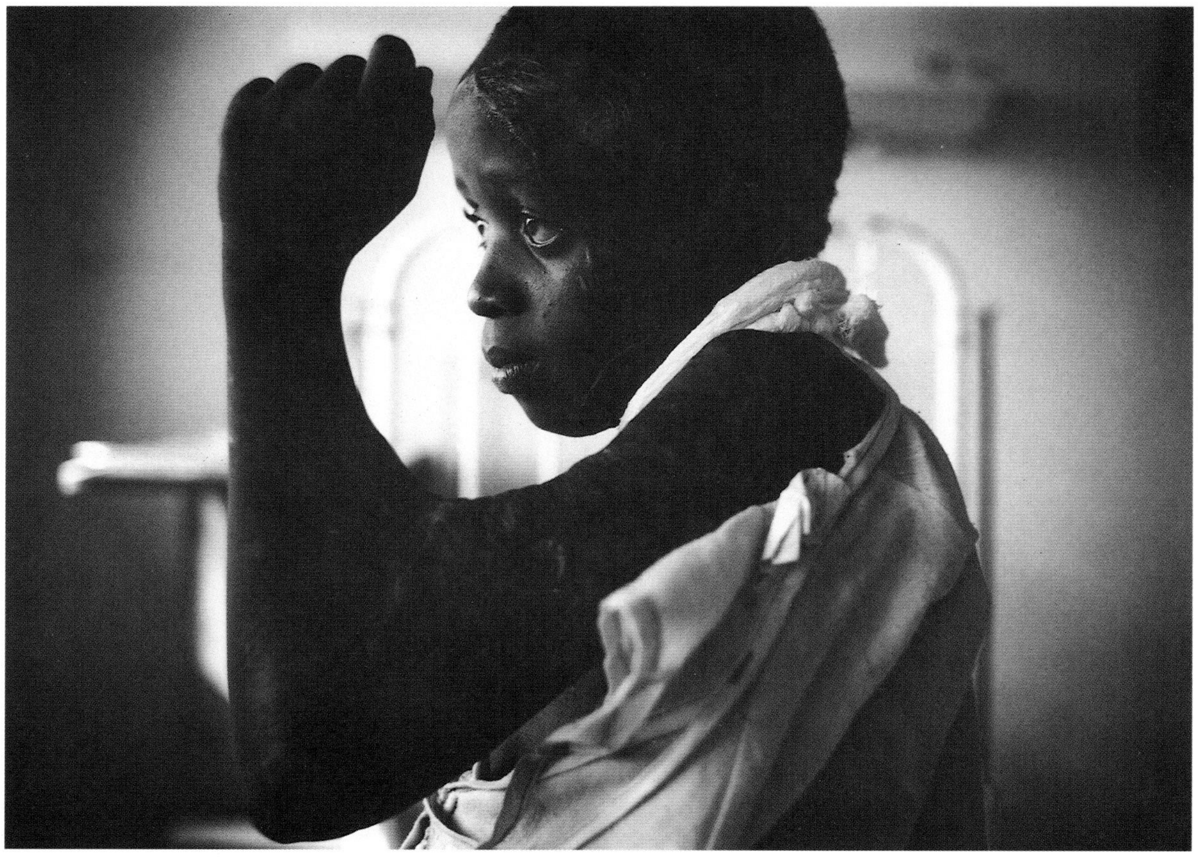

burn ward, Nairobi

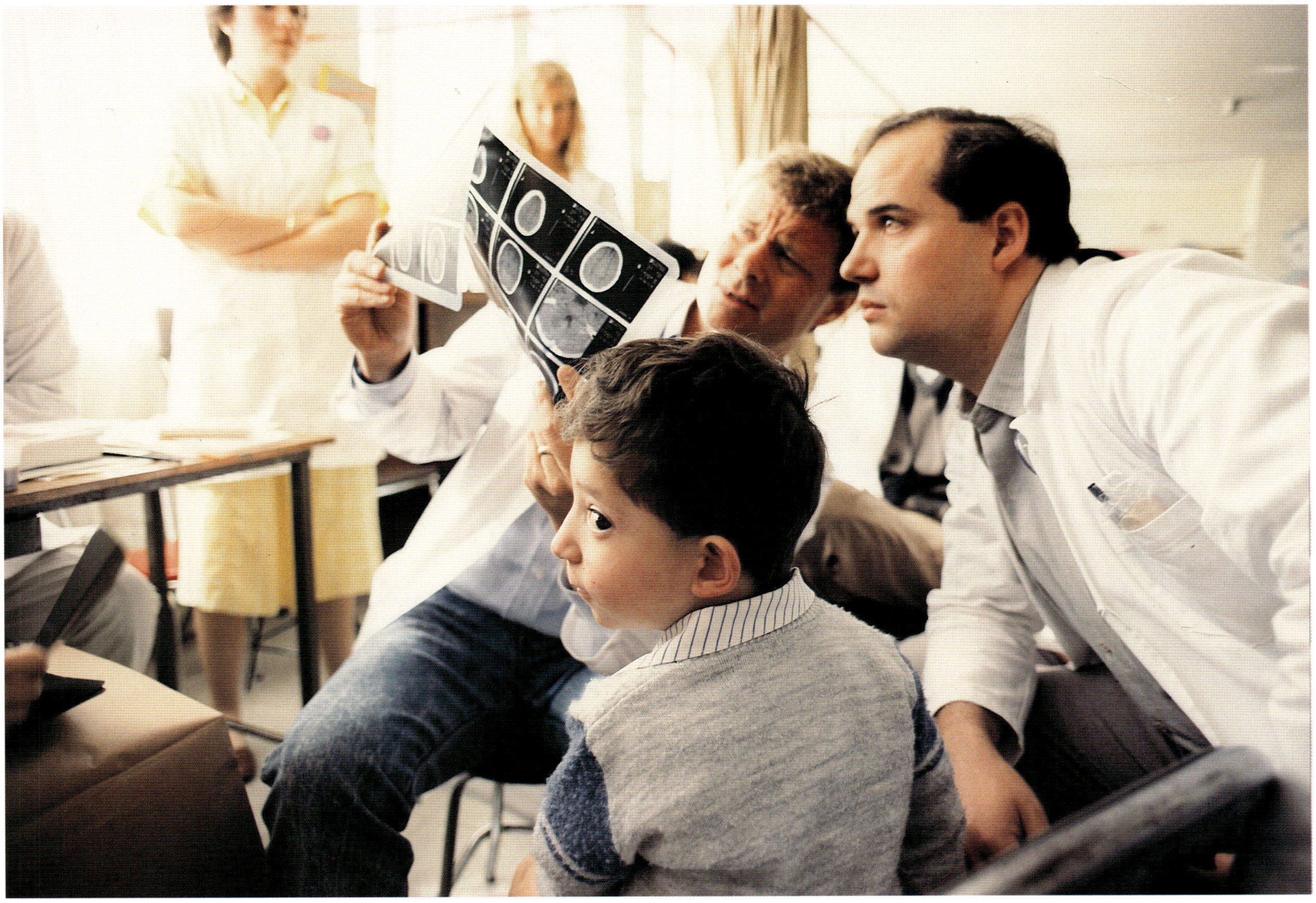

patient in screening, Manizales

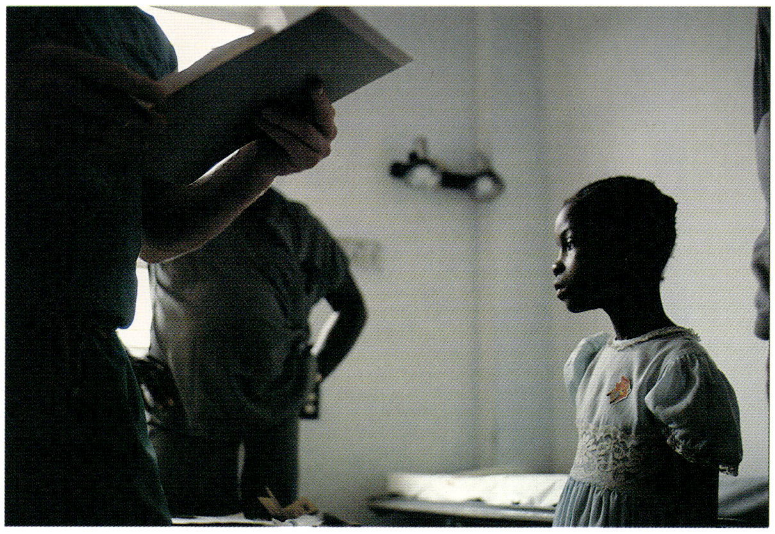

patient in screening, Monrovia

This voluntary and humane service
has been extremely beneficial to Ghana
and has put smiles on the faces of many young Ghanaians
who would otherwise have been doomed to an unhappy existence.

THE HONORABLE ERIC K. OTOO
GHANAIAN AMBASSADOR TO THE UNITED STATES

burn ward, Nairobi

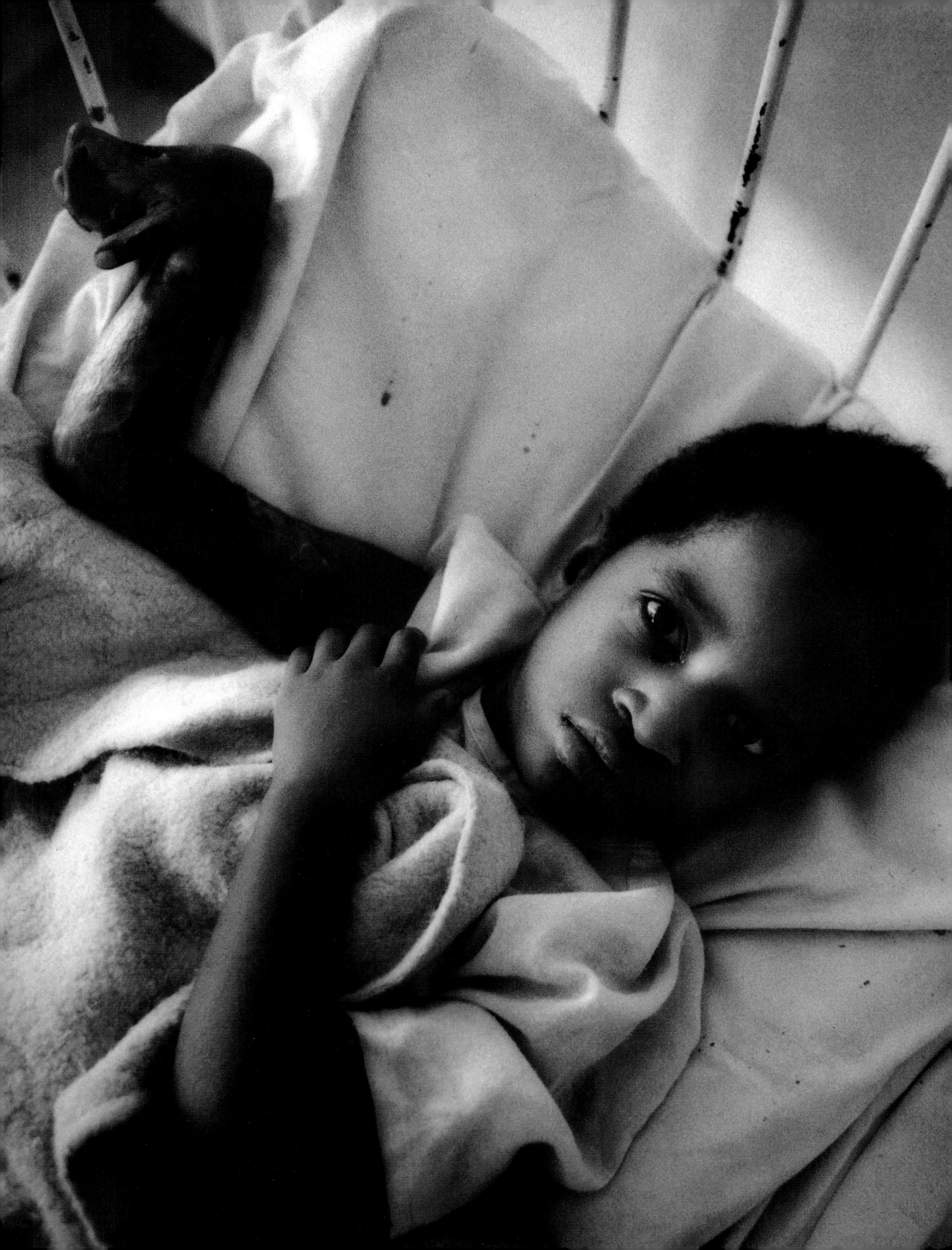

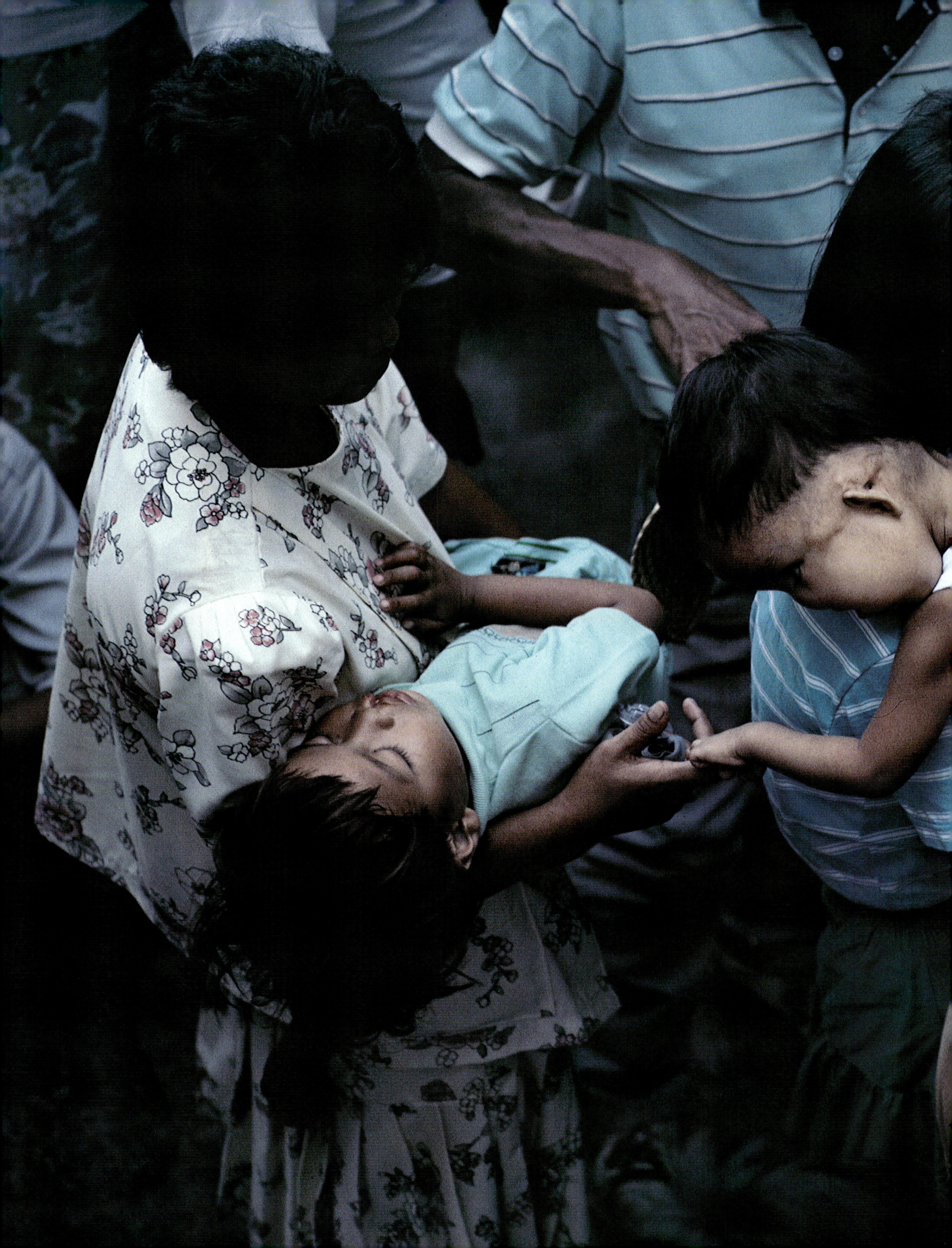

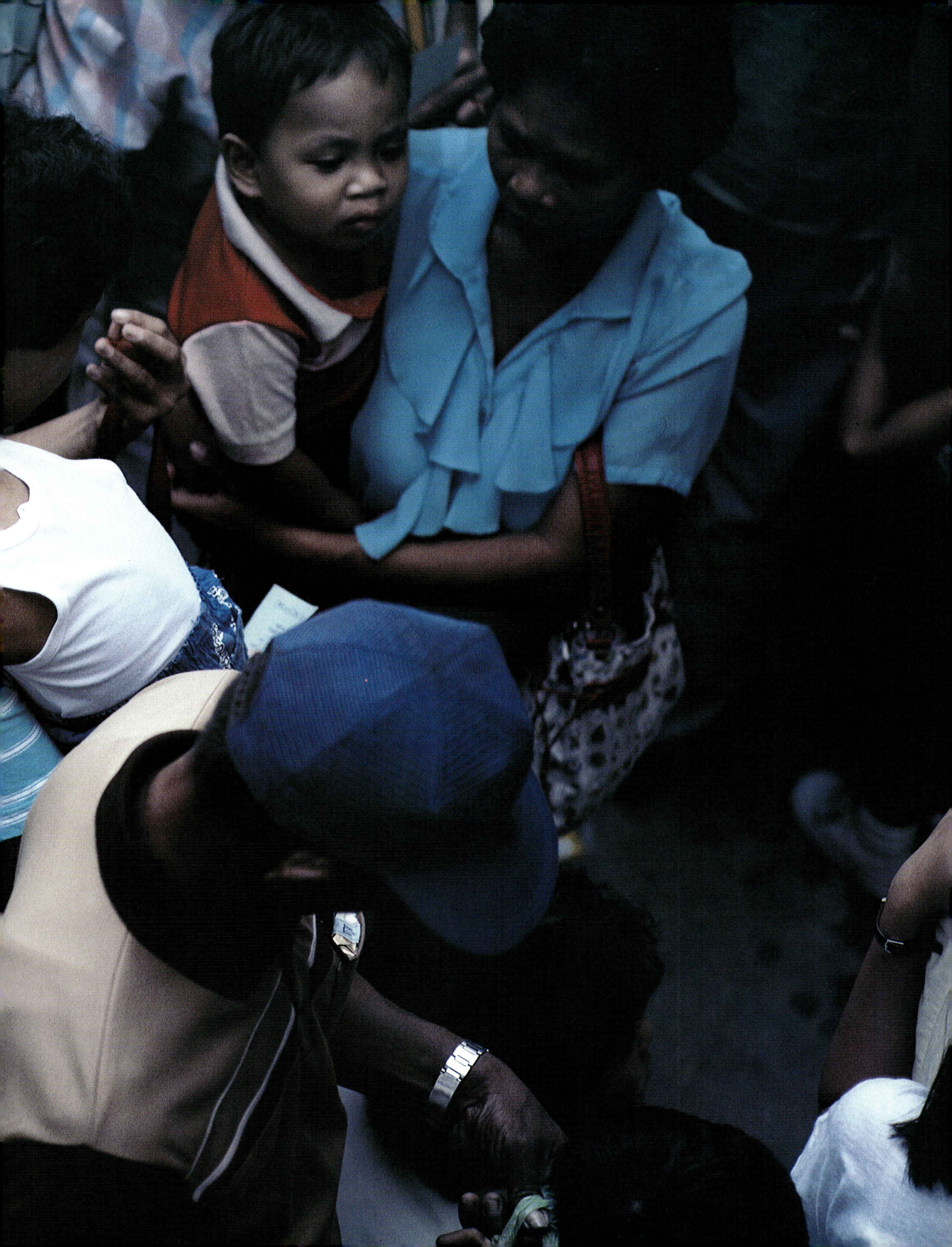

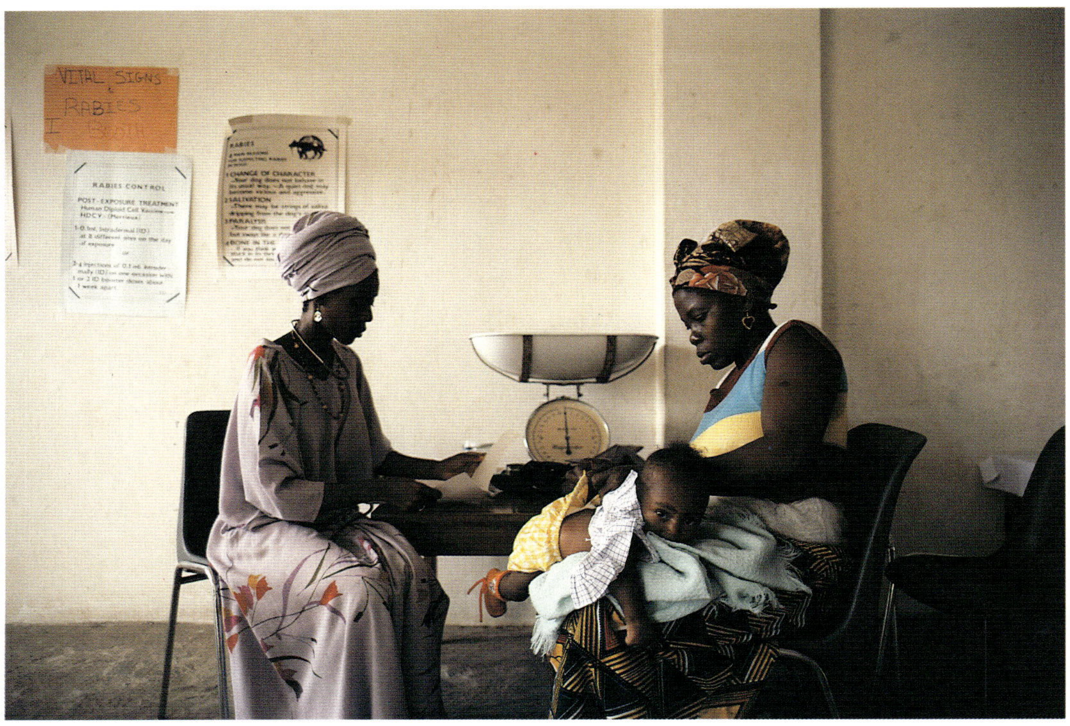

patient screening, Monrovia
(previous spread) families wait for screening, Manila

There was one bed, however, where a boy
about five years old was alone. He had no father.
His mother had died days before his arrival.
He had a cleft palate.
What made this boy stand out among the other children,
was the fact that he had no one with him
and despite his deformity
he always had a smile in his eyes.

His chart showed that he had come to the hospital alone.
I held his hand as he was prepared for surgery,
and told him that it was his mother's hand
holding him through me.

ALAIN DICK
OSI VOLUNTEER

pre-op ward, Naga City

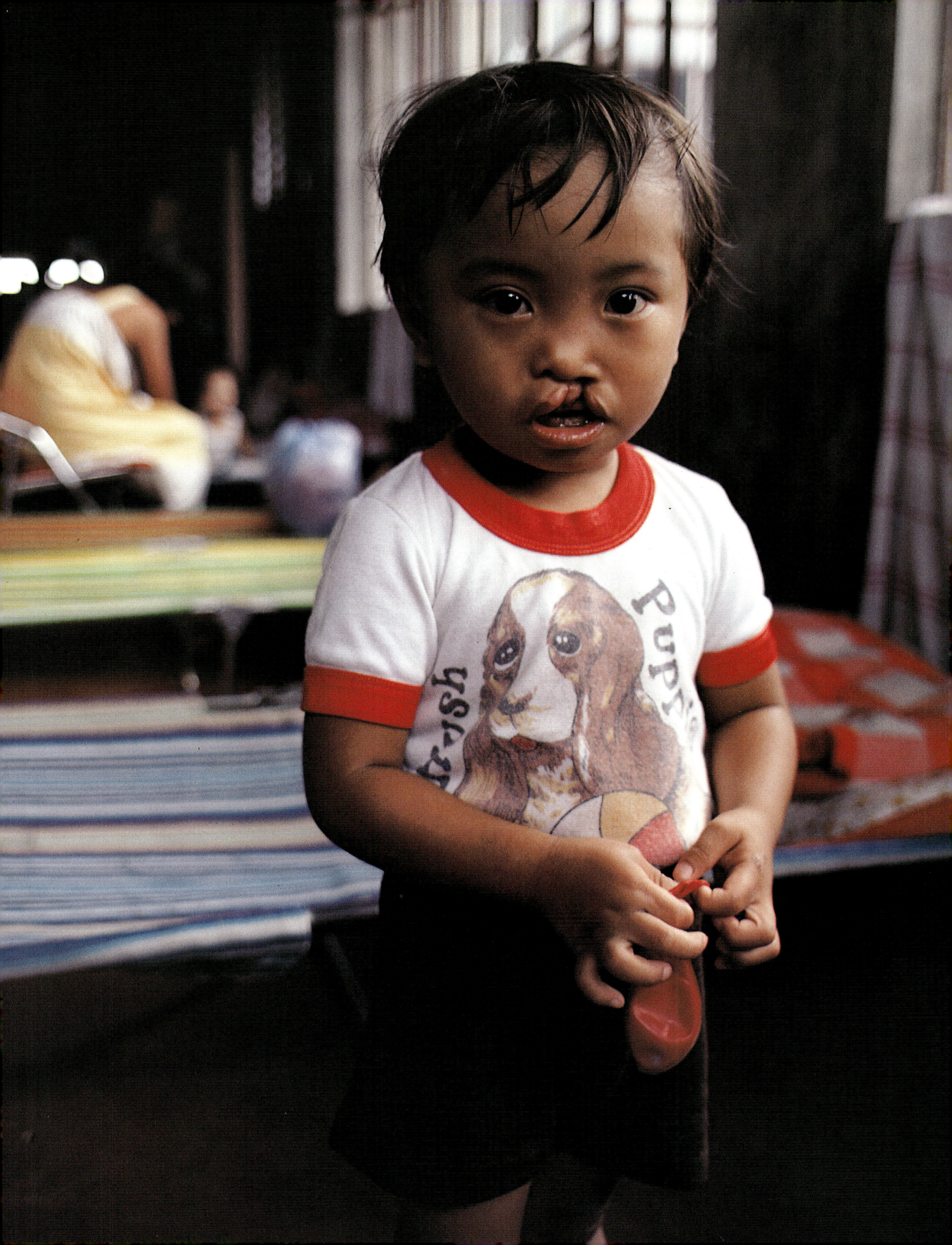

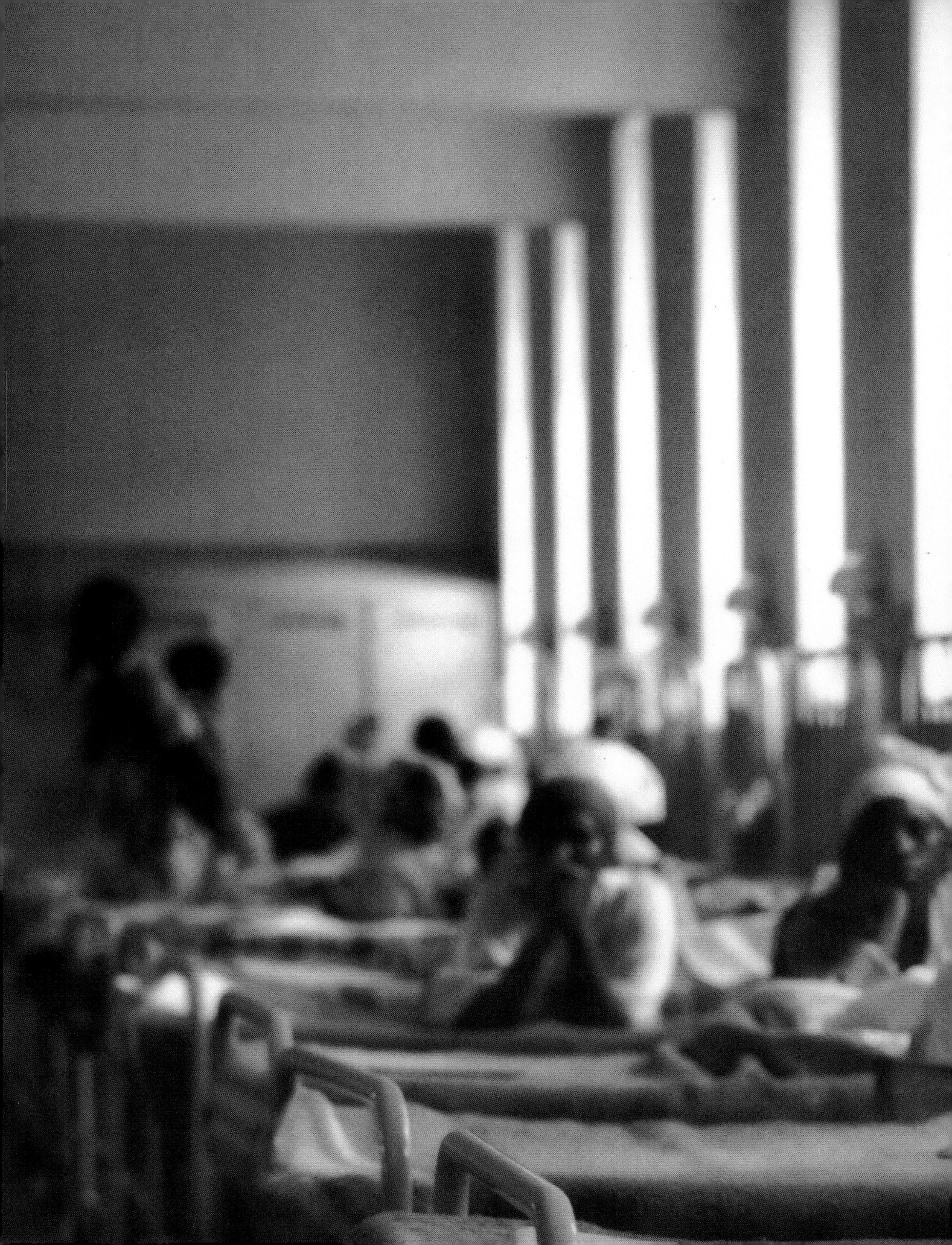

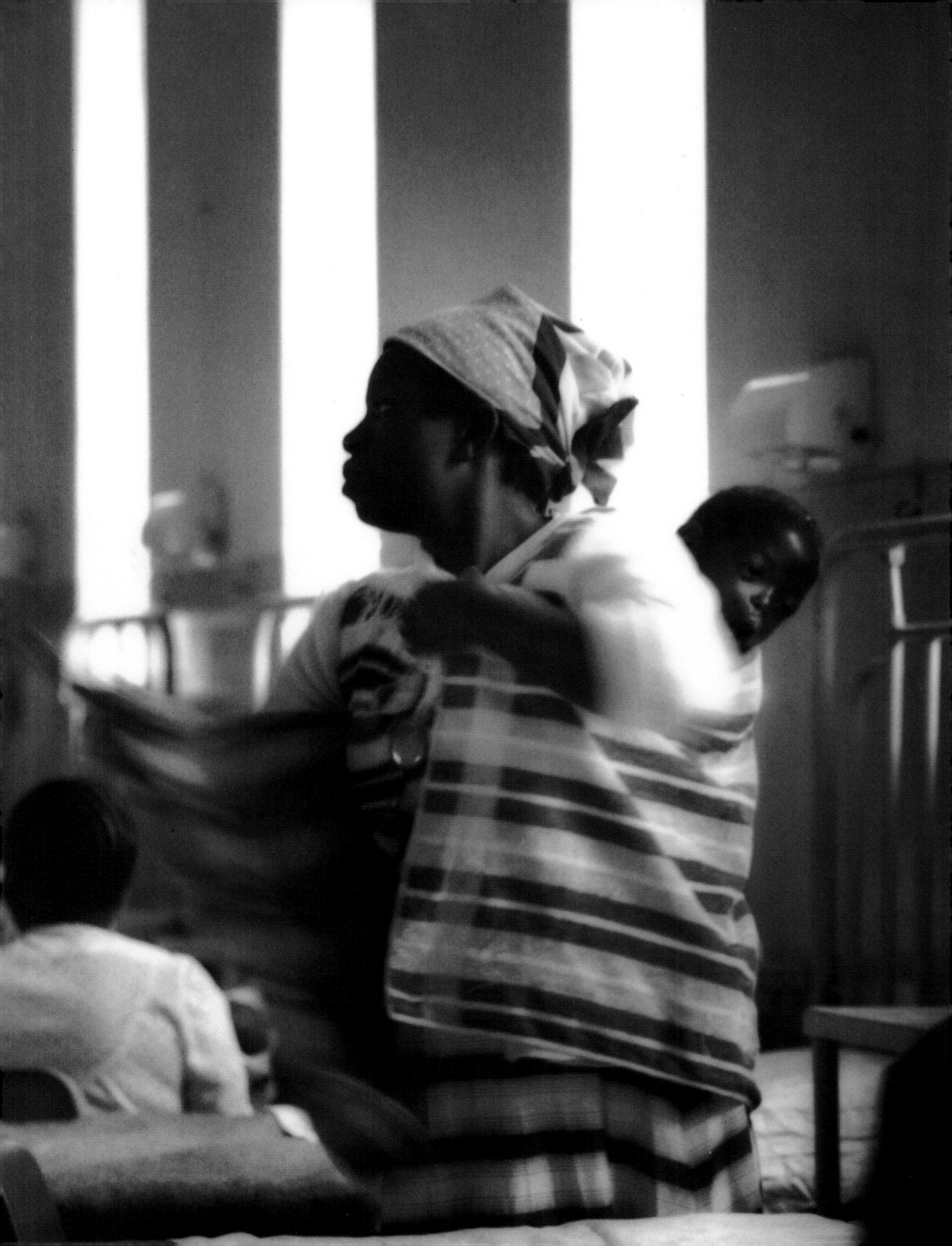

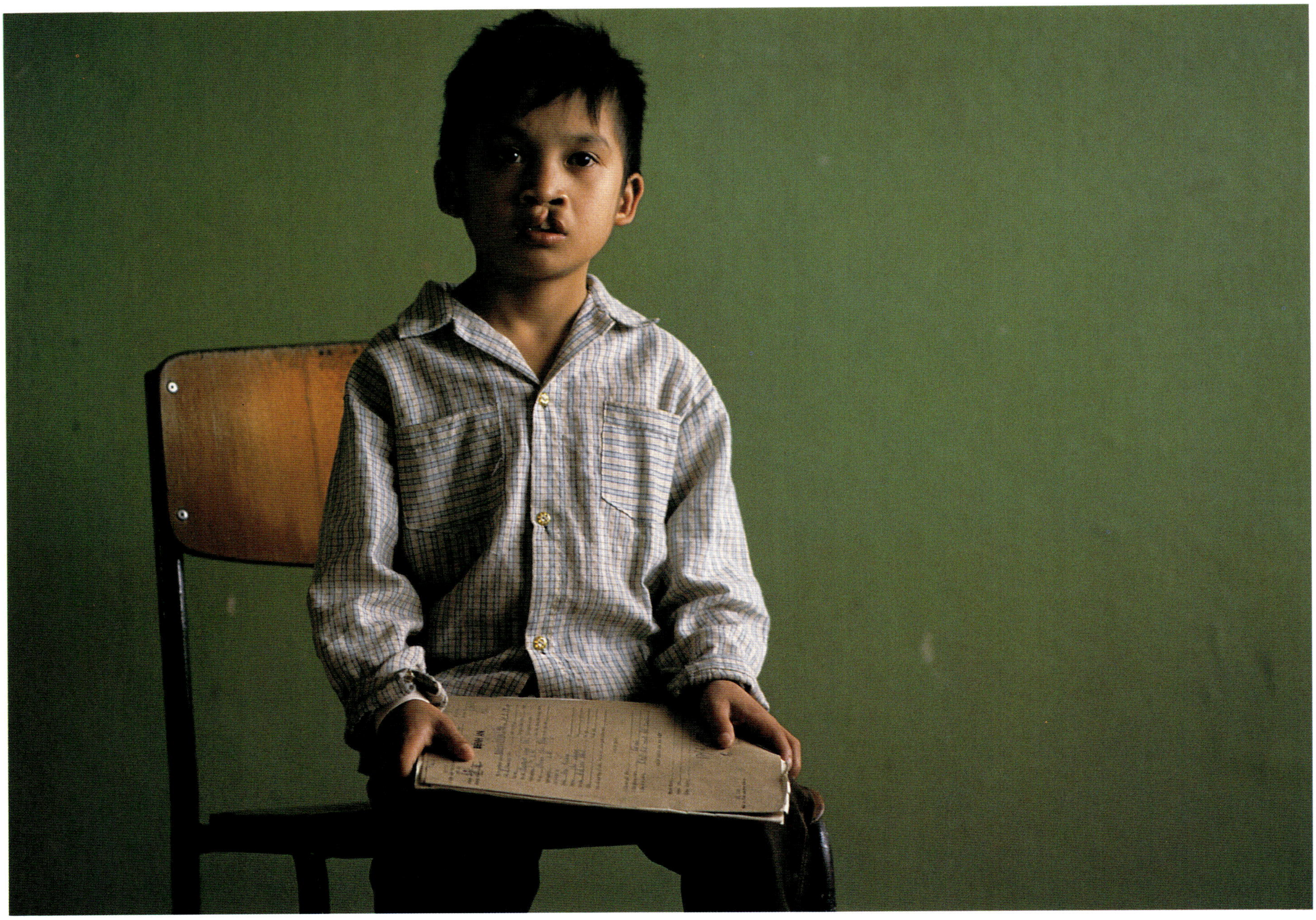

patient in screening, Saigon
(previous spread) families and patients on children's ward, Nairobi

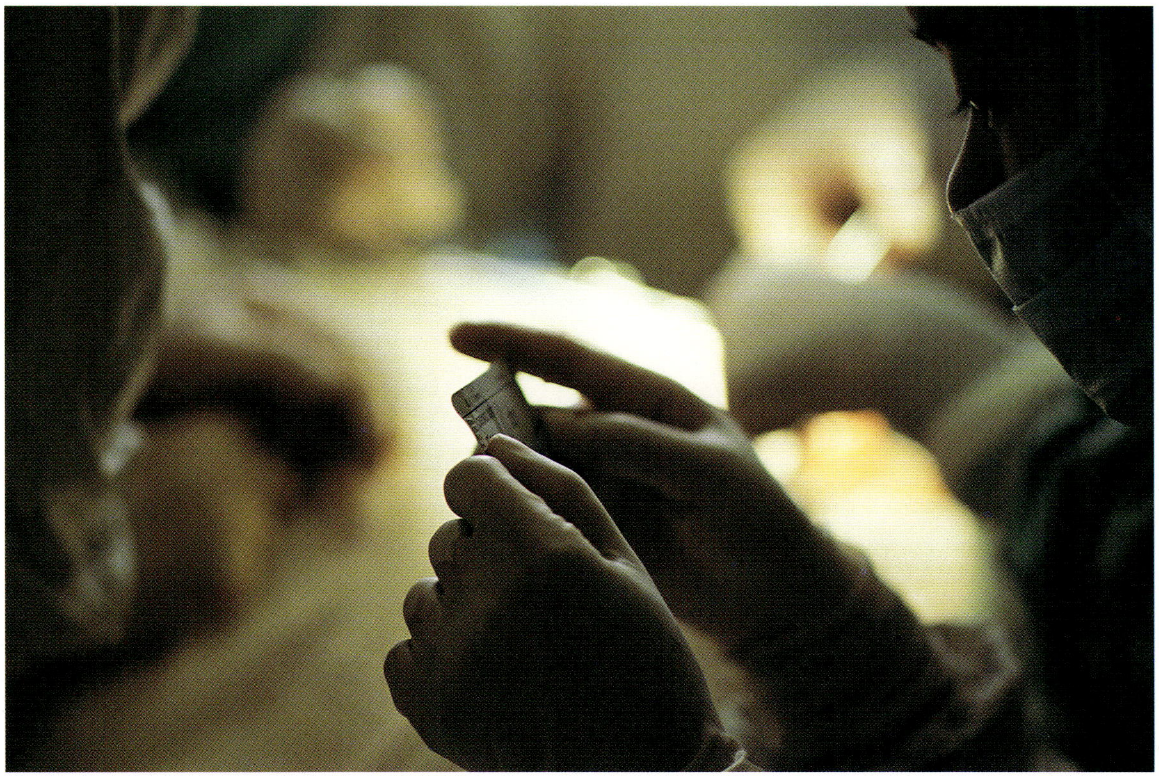

surgery, Panama City

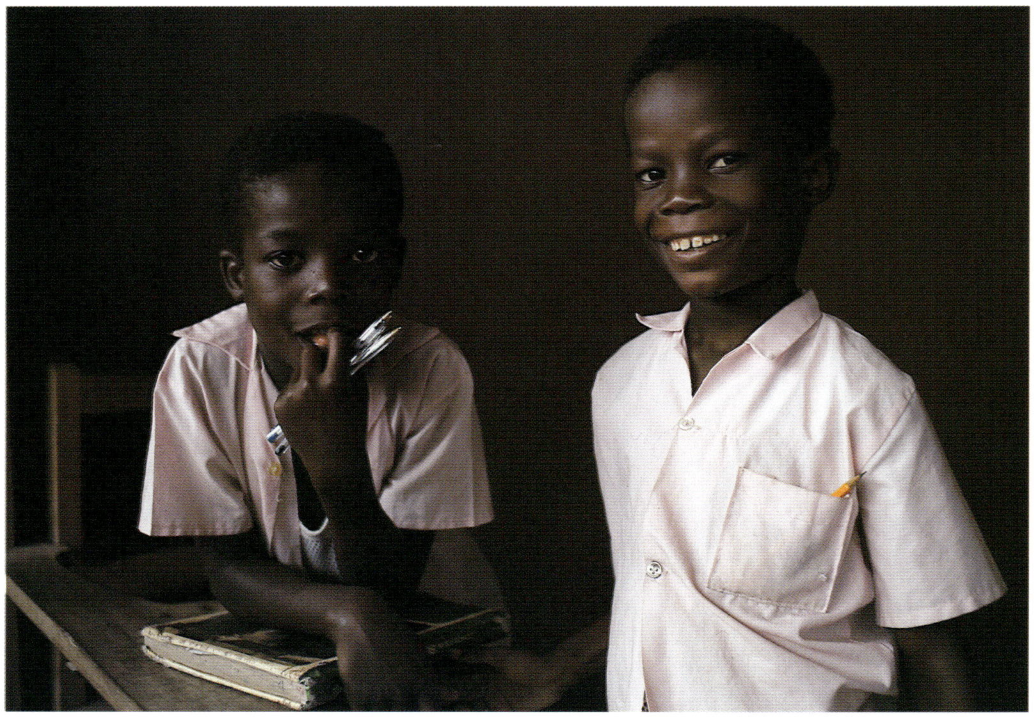

school boys, Monrovia

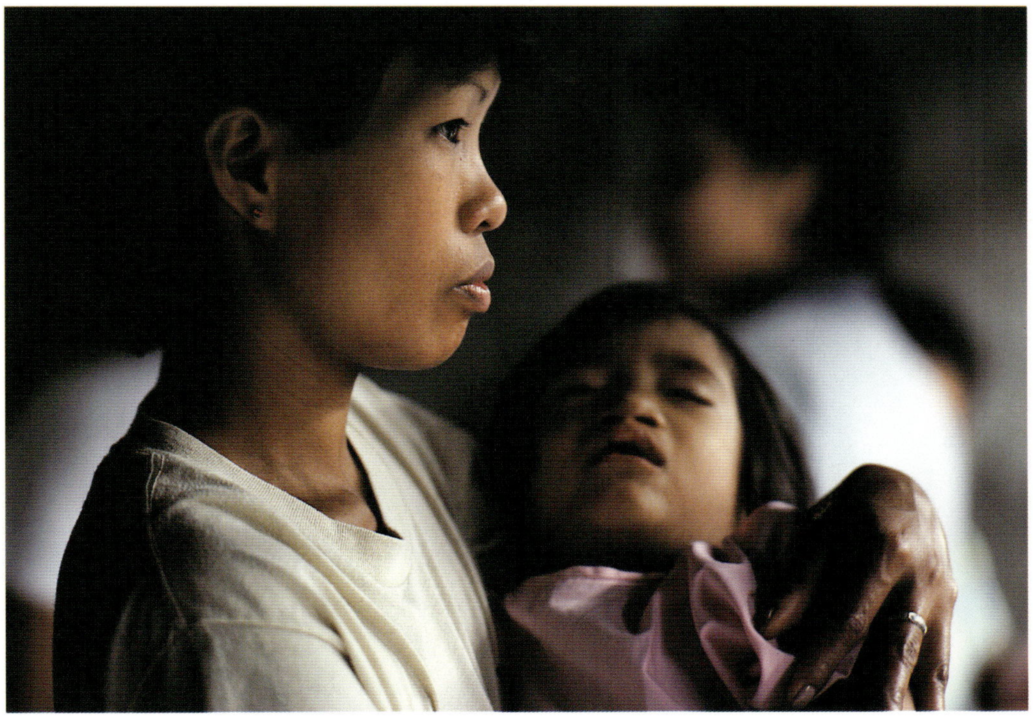

mother and child, Naga City

We had the privilage to observe a humanitarian group working like an army of ants with the most powerful arms, those of universal love, and this has filled our lives with light.

To be close to a child's pain and change it to a smile is to be close to the doors of heaven.

SERGIO, JULIA, AND VIRGINIA JAEN
PANAMA CITY, PANAMA

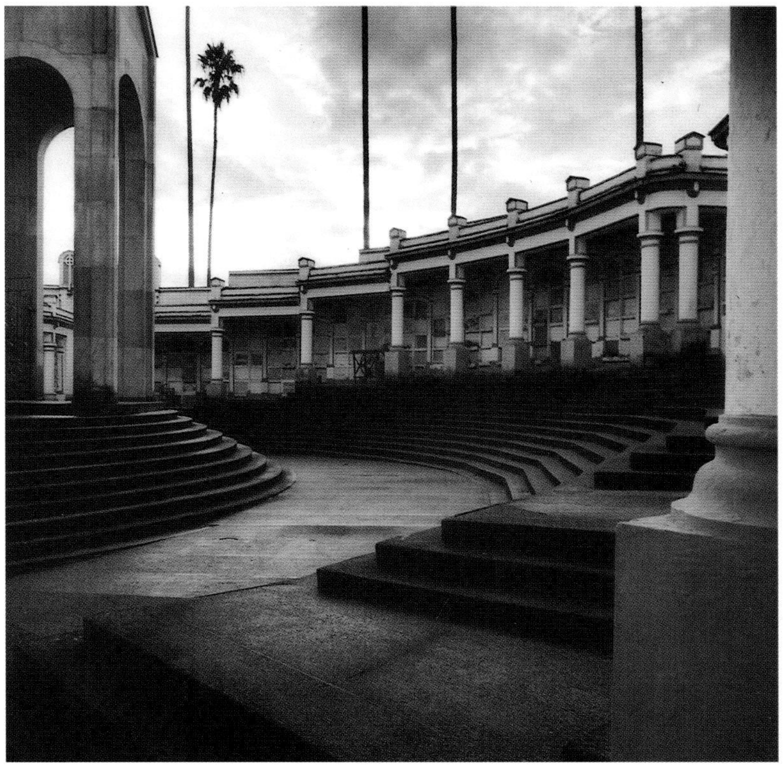

Manizales

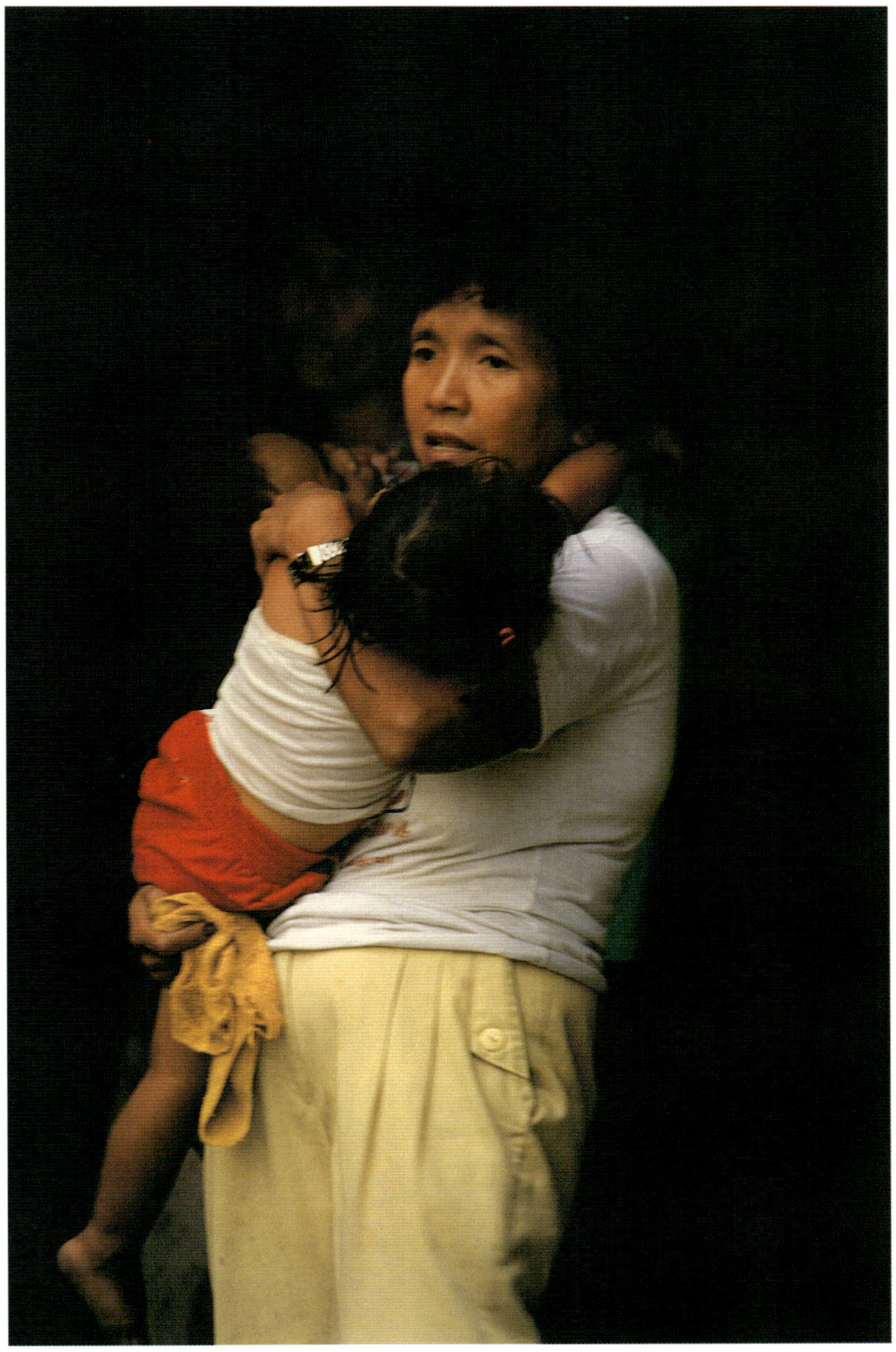

waiting in screening, Manila

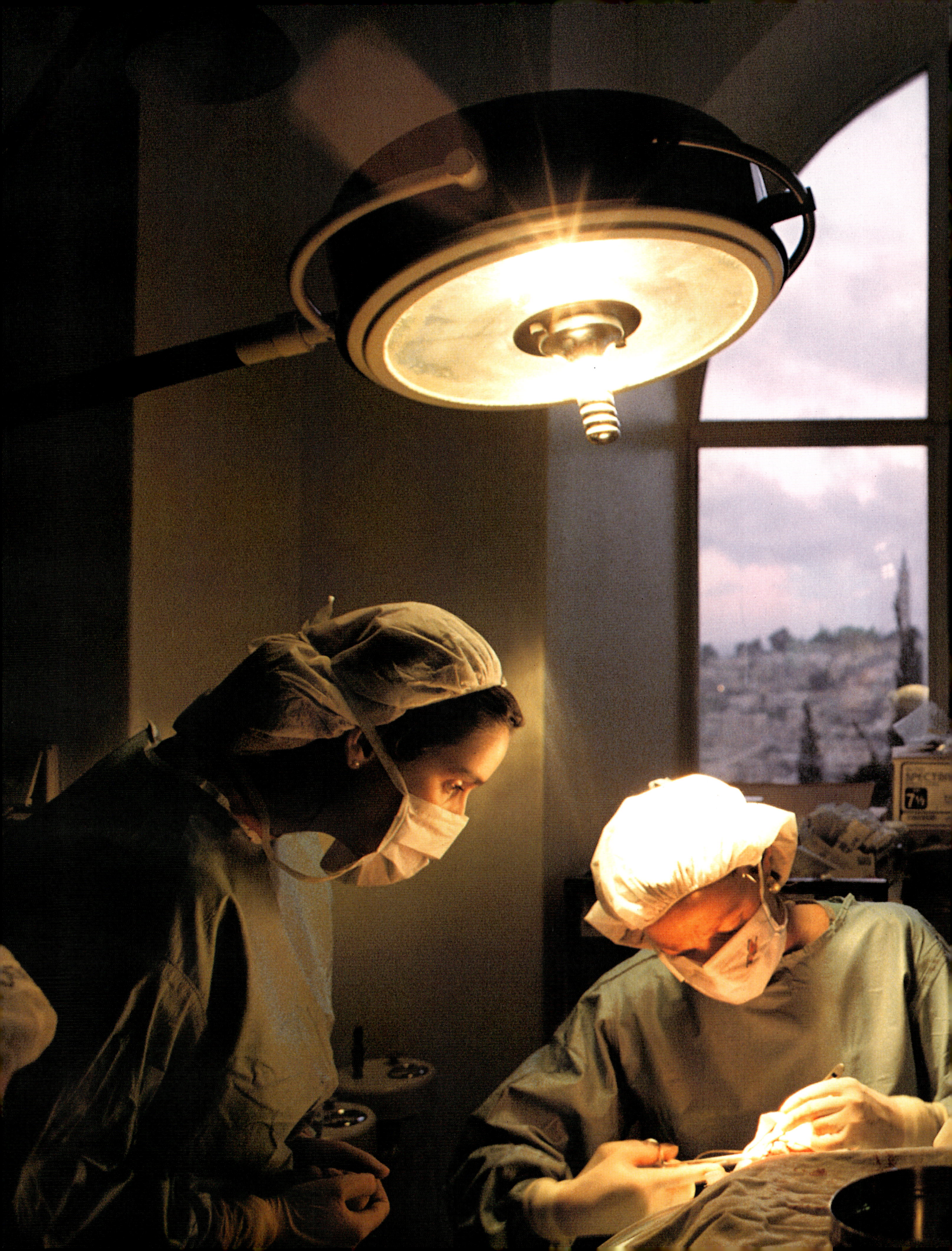

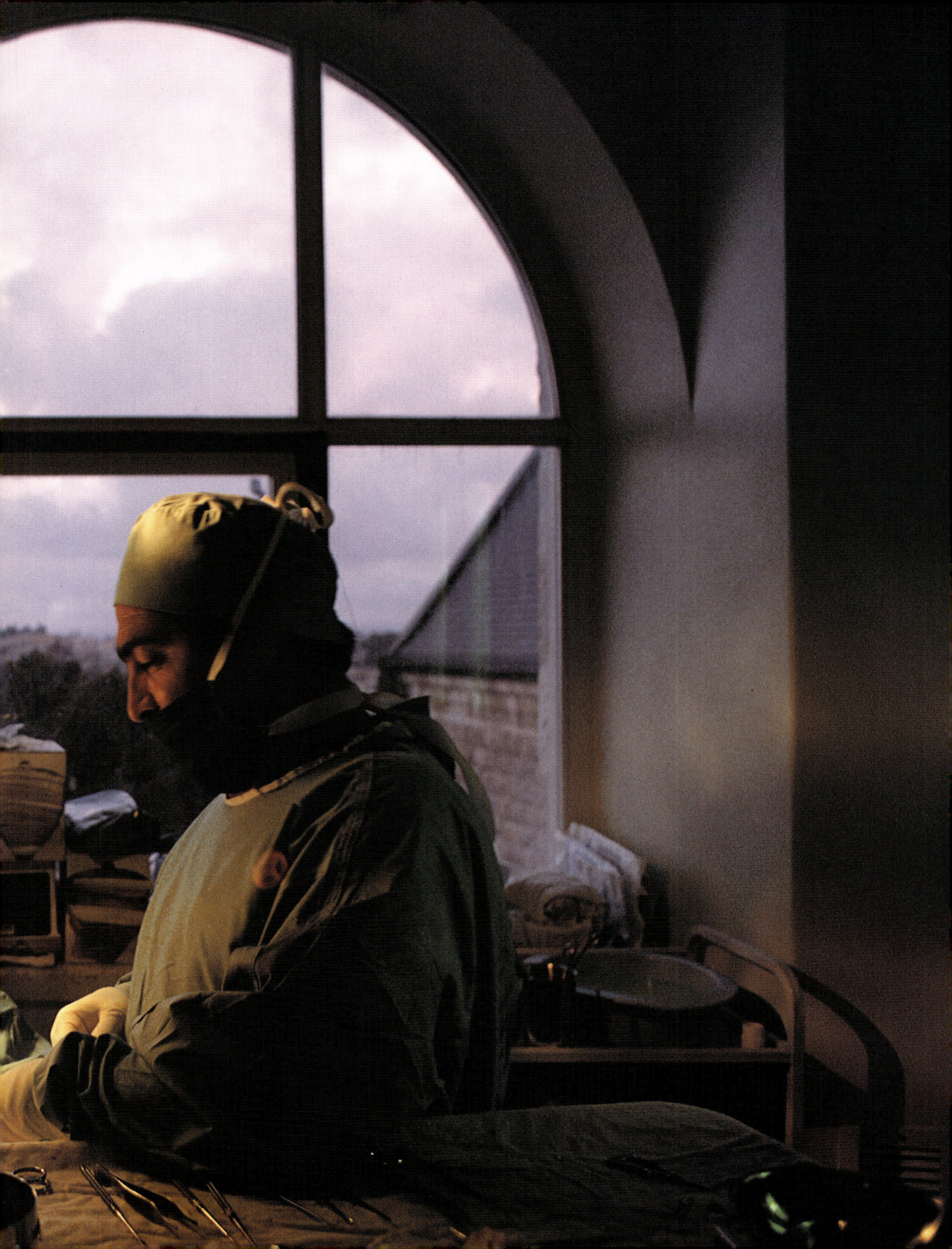

(previous spread) evening surgery, Jerusalem

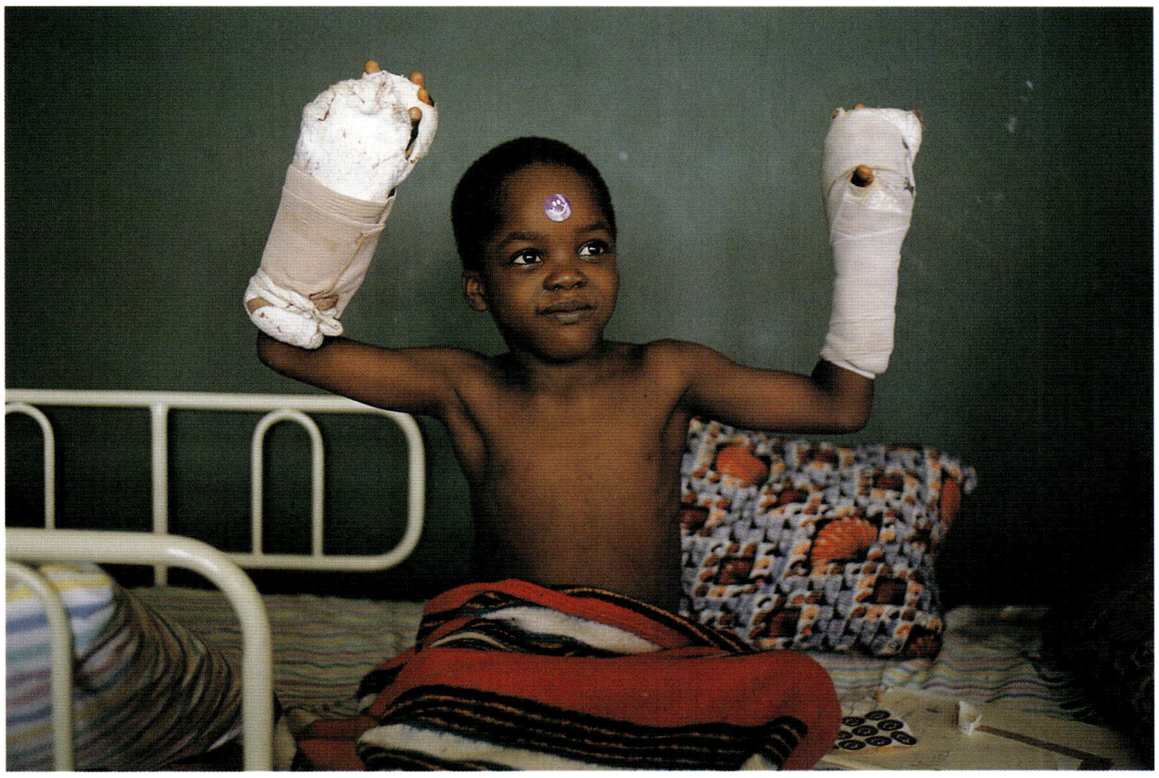

patient in post-op, Monrovia

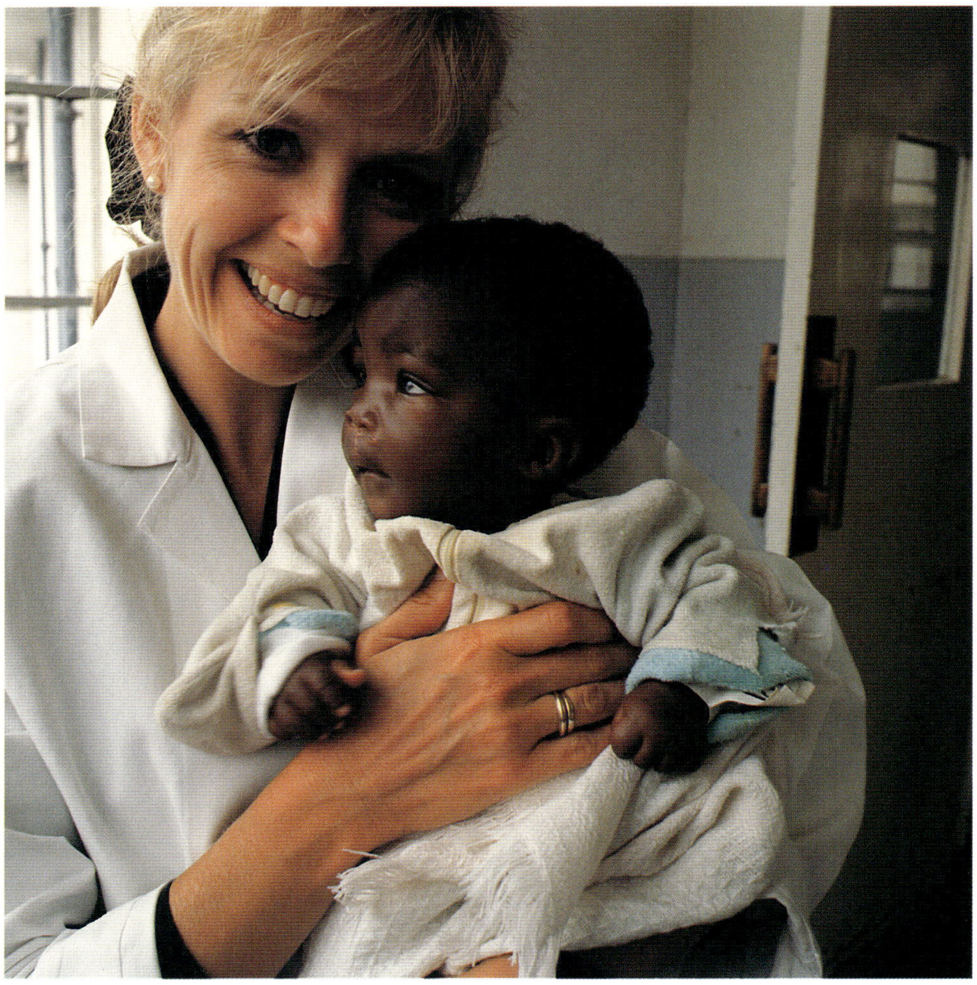

volunteer and patient, Nairobi
photograph by Barbara Kinney

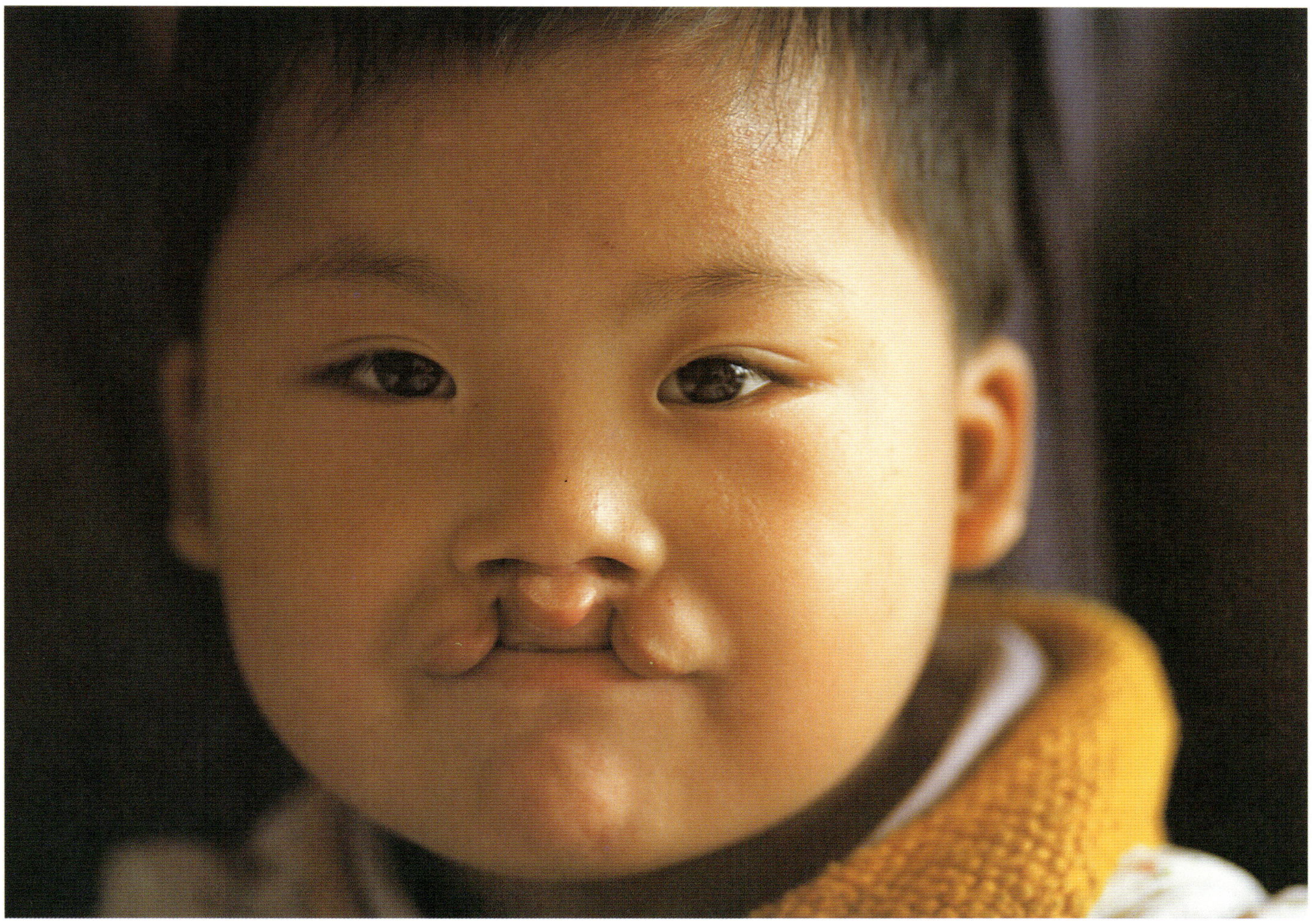

patient with cleft lip and palate, Hangzhou

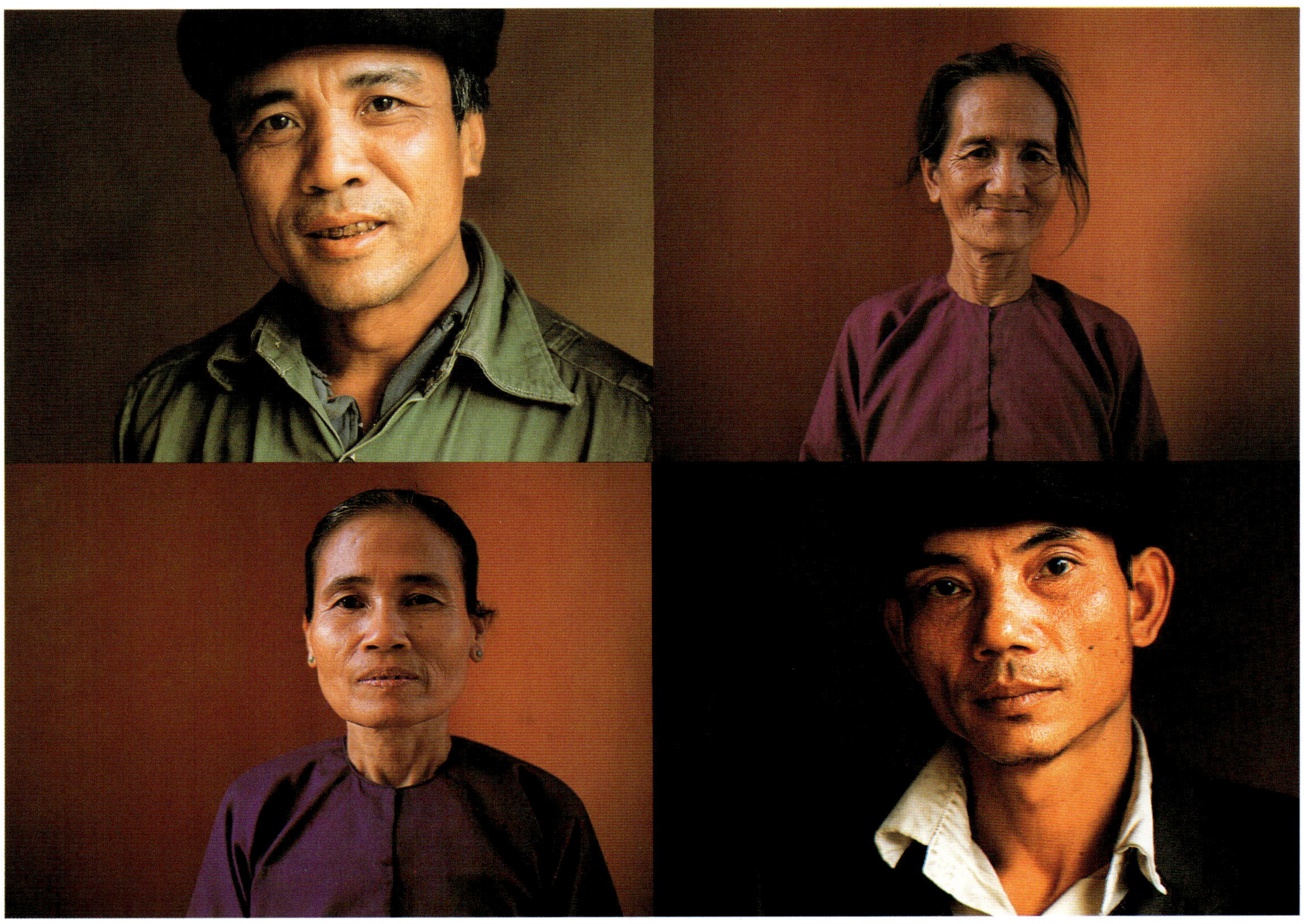

parents at hospital, Saigon

Great ideas begin with simple acts of action.
What nations are sometimes unable to accomplish
may be approachable by individuals
who embrace what is shared in common
rather than what divides us.

Operation Smile concentrates on a common denominator of human existence;
the love of a child,
and a prayer for a hopeful future.

MICHAEL MAGEE, MD
OSI MEDICAL VOLUNTEER

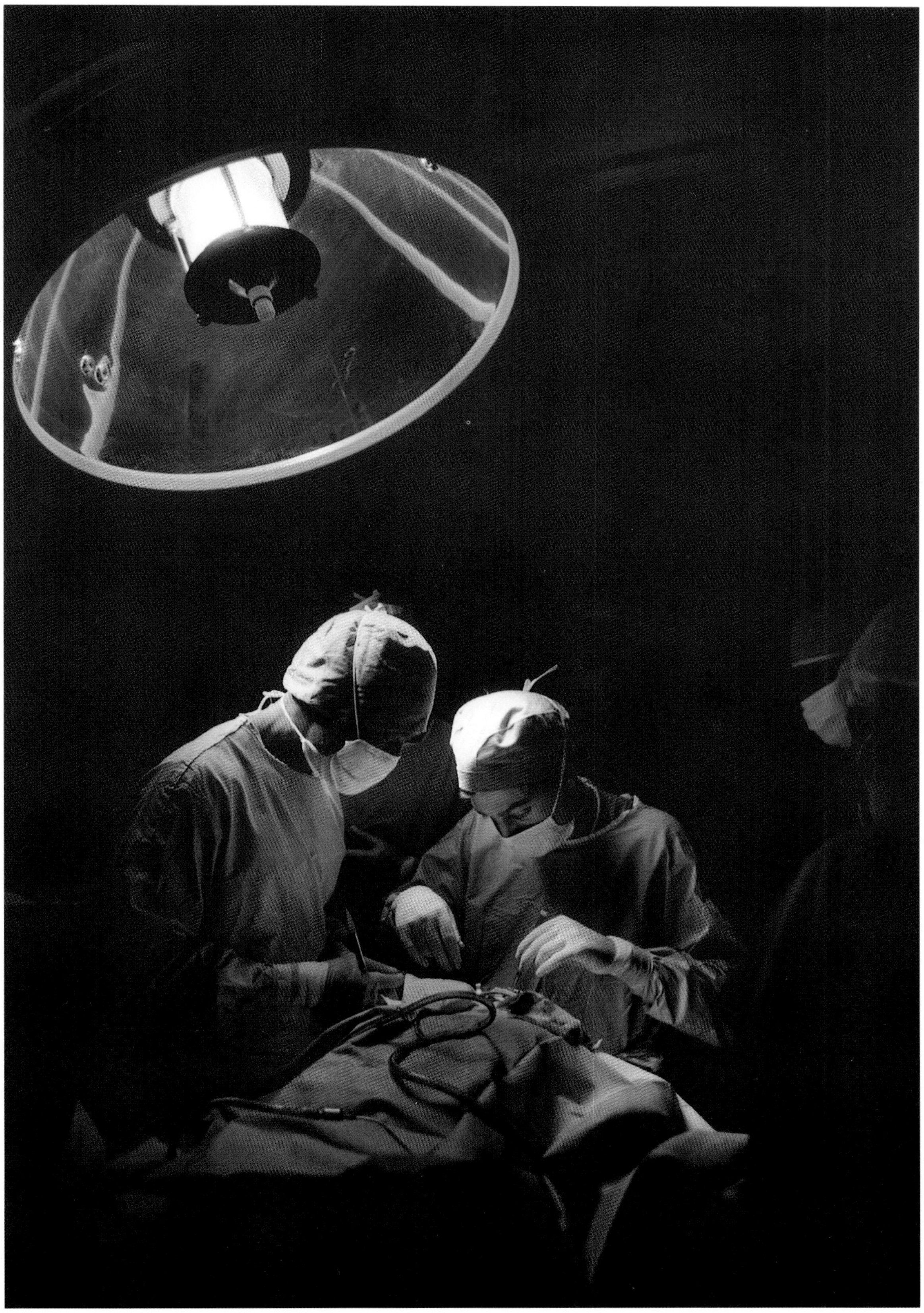

surgery, Manizales

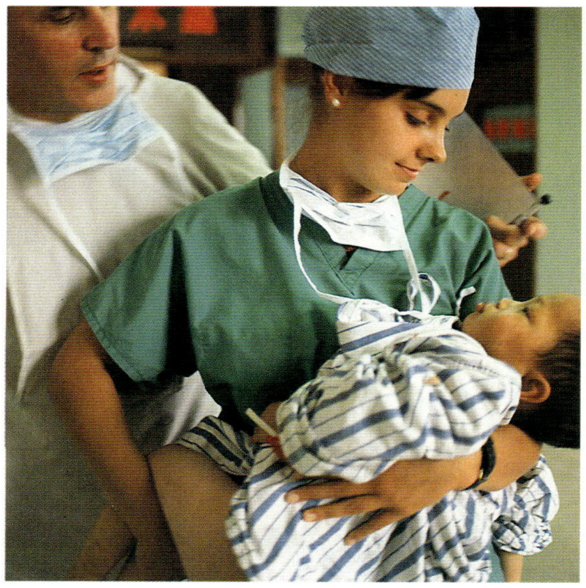

teenage volunteer and patient, Hangzhou
patient before scar revision and palate surgery, Monrovia

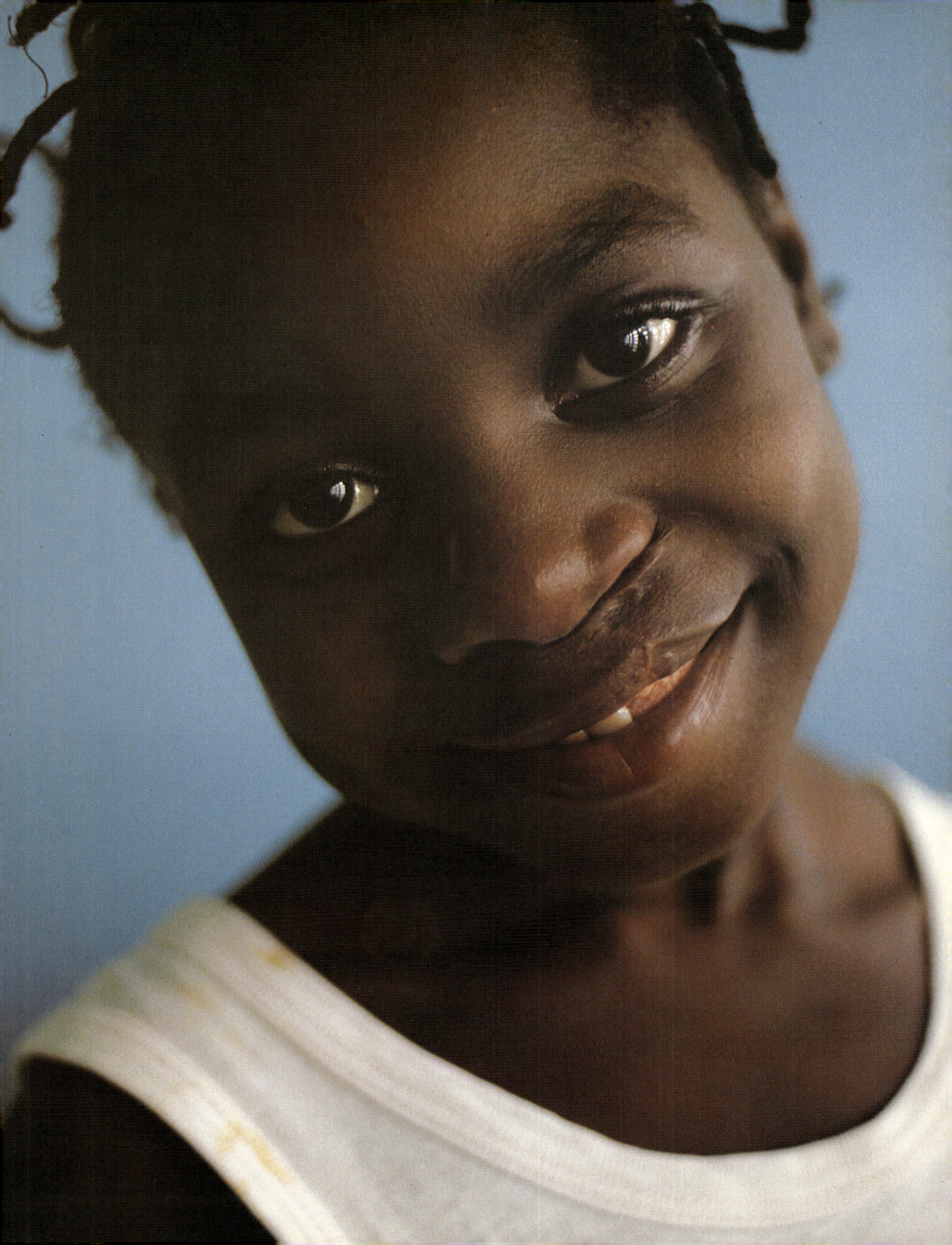

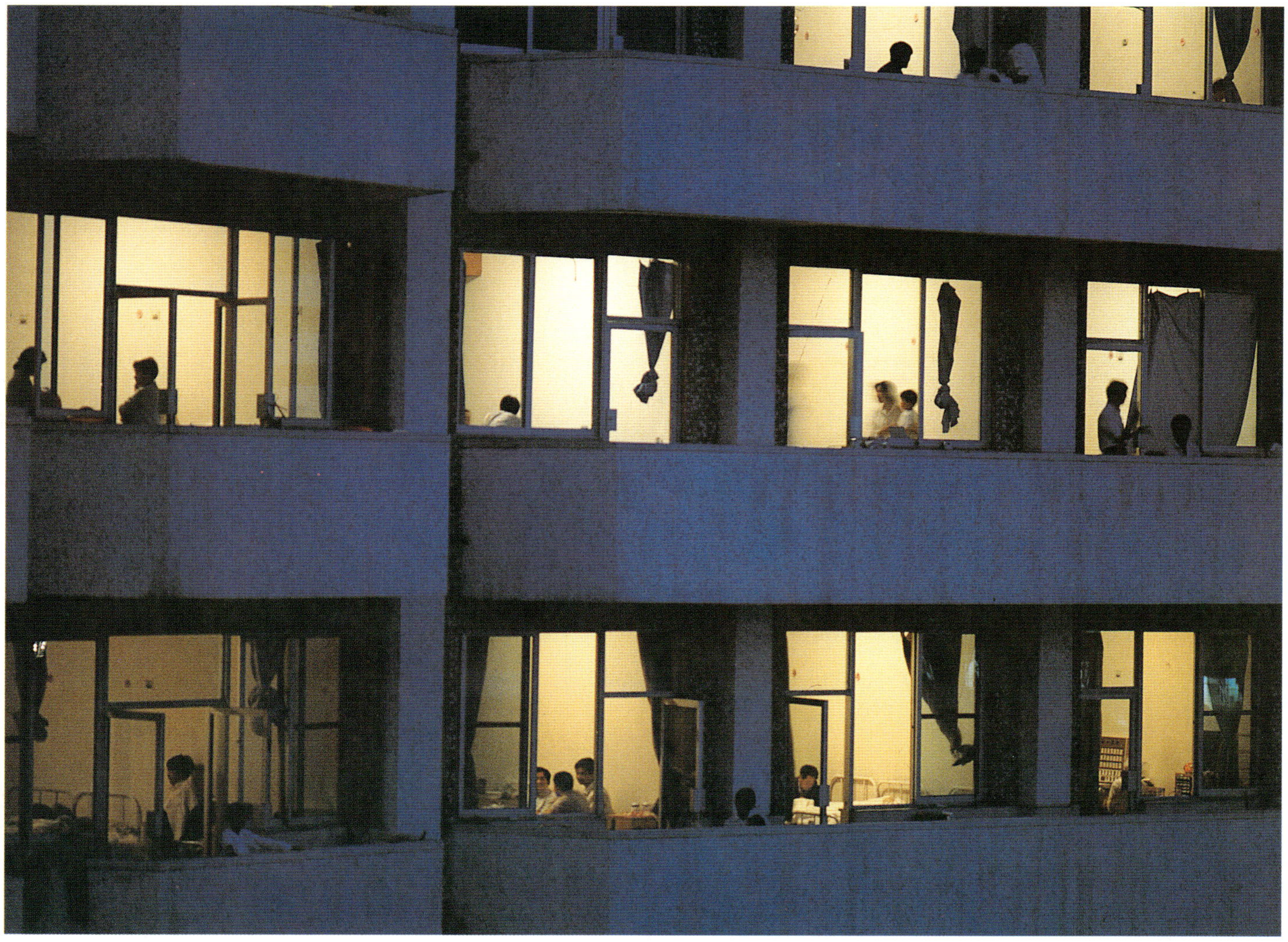

dusk at hospital for plastic surgery, Hangzhou

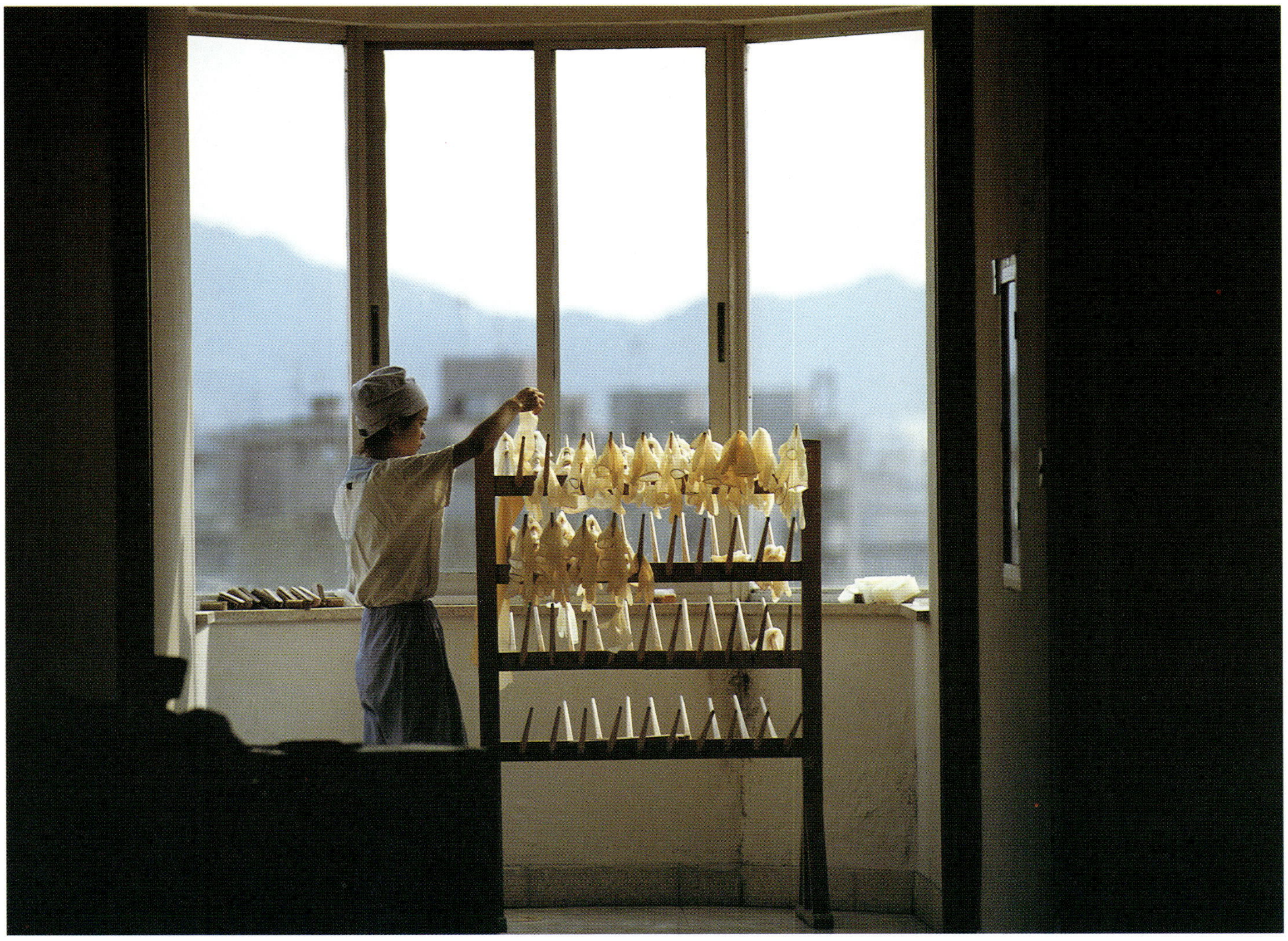

nurse hangs surgical gloves, sterilized for reuse, Hangzhou

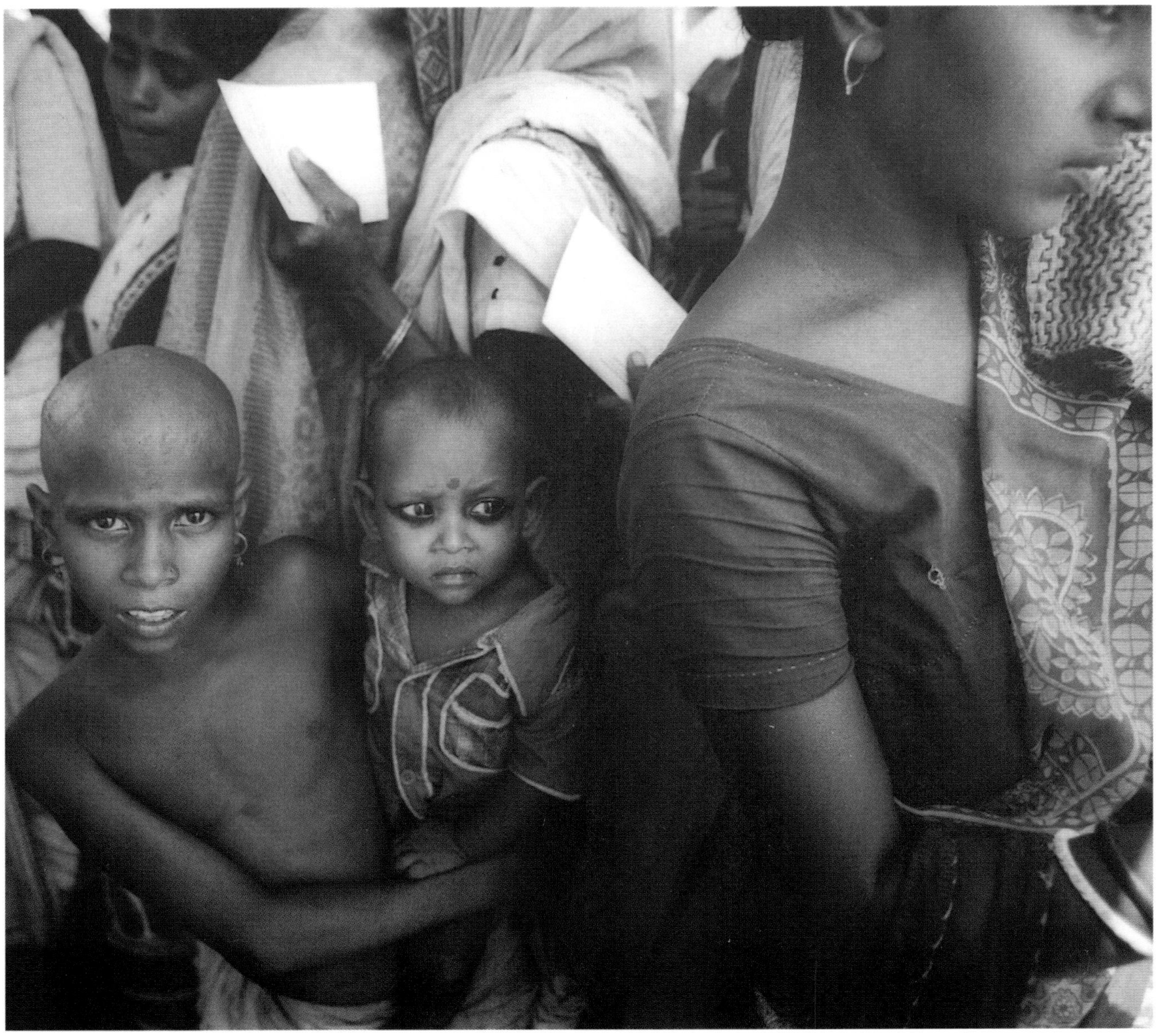

children at feeding center, Calcutta

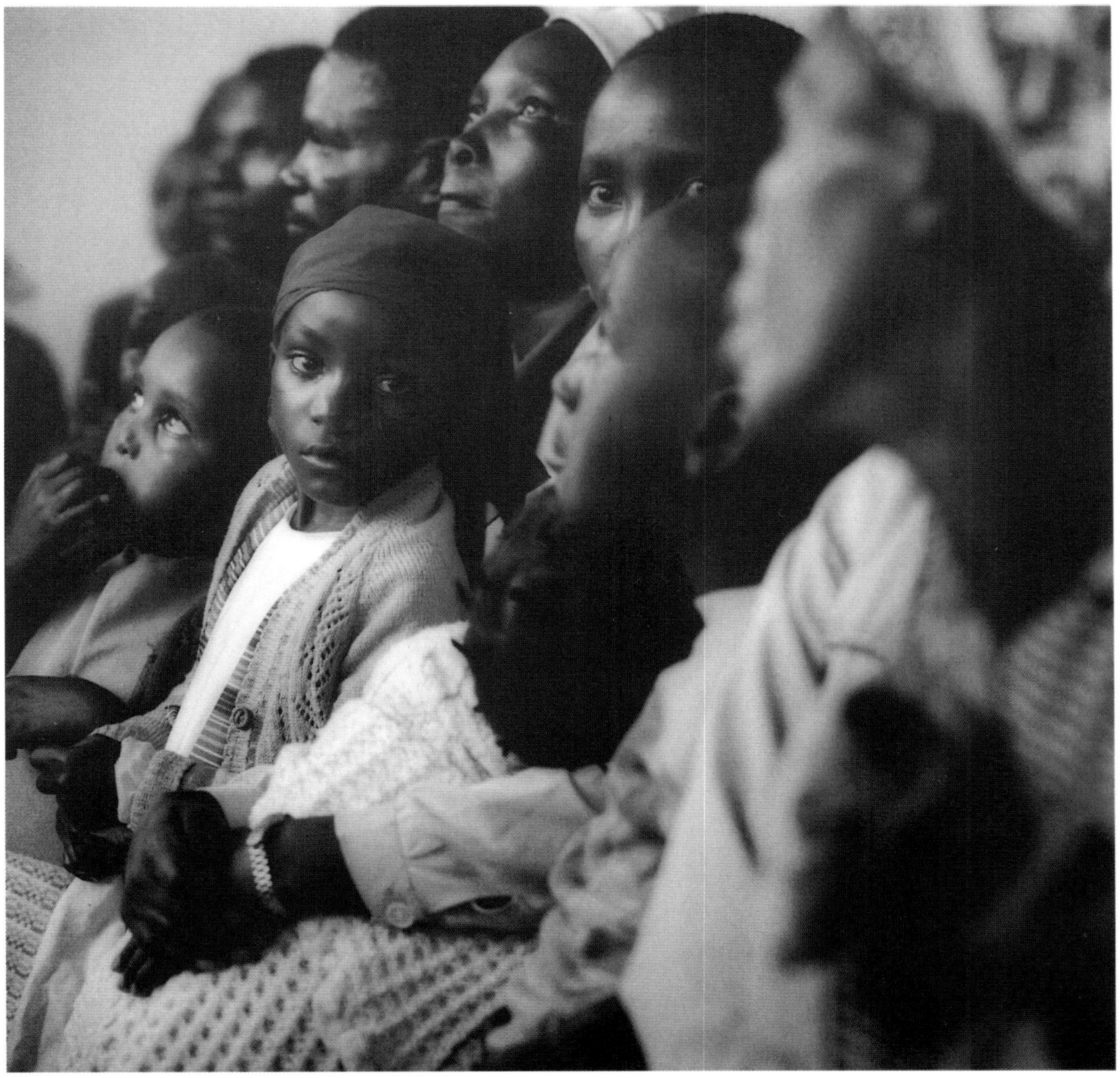

families await screening, Nairobi

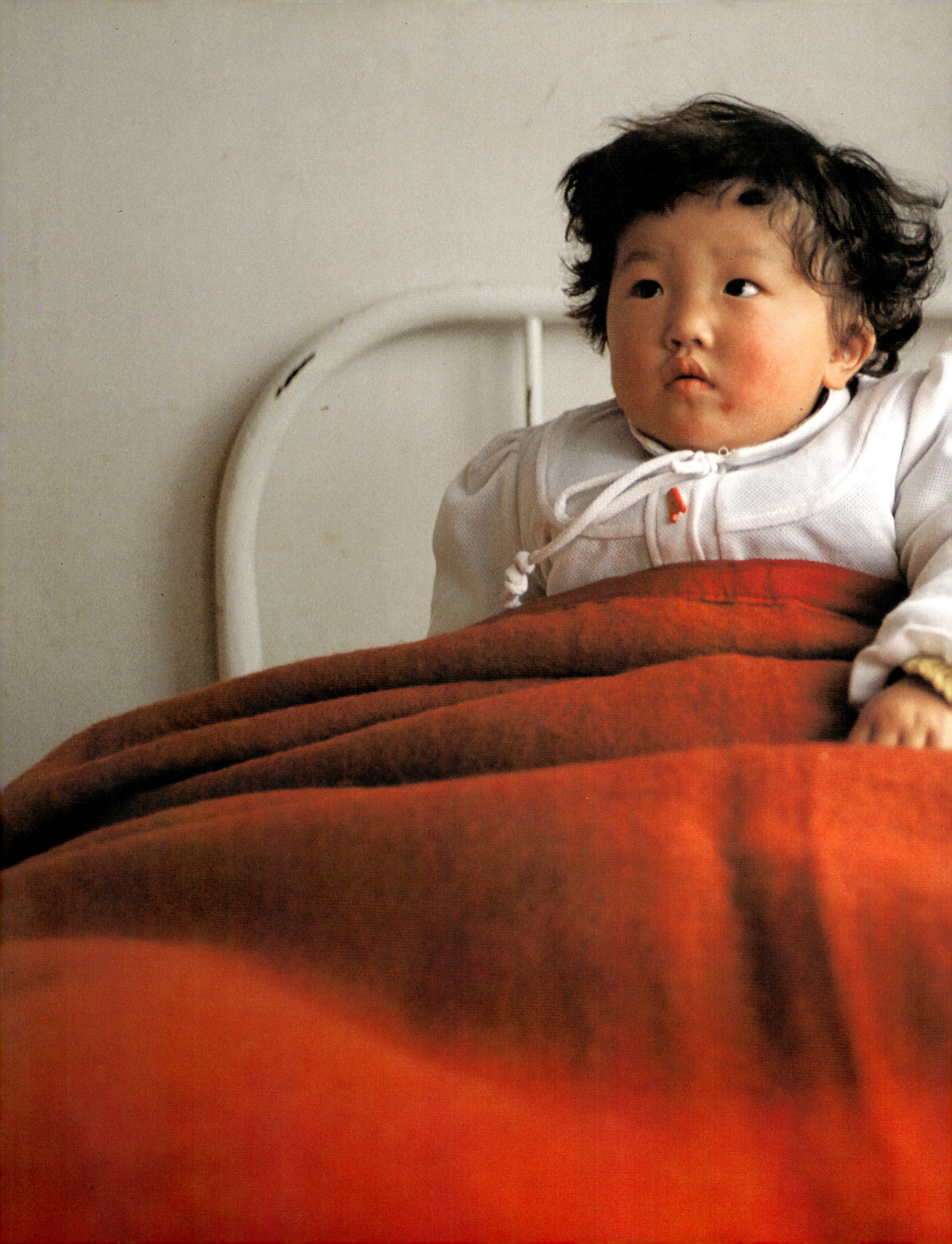

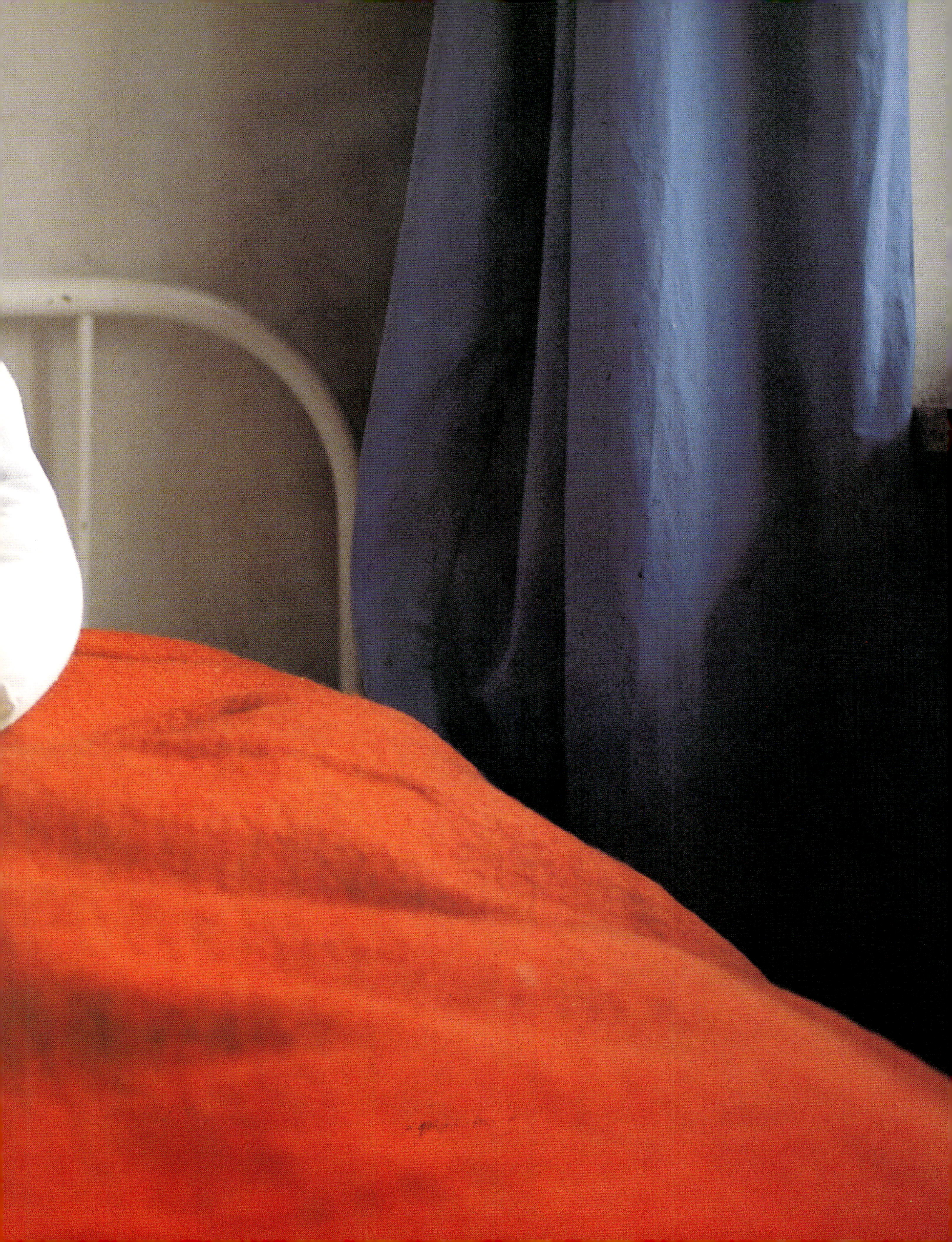

(previous spread) patient on children's ward, Hangzhou

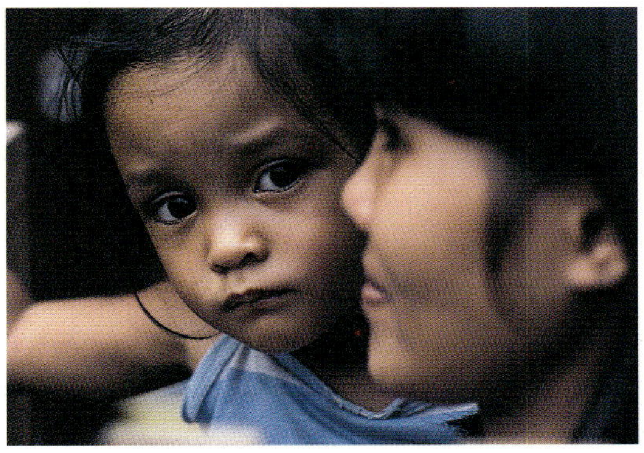

I shall never forget the broken faces looking up at us in front of the screening clinic on that first day.

MORTON H. GOLDSTEIN, MD
OSI MEDICAL VOLUNTEER

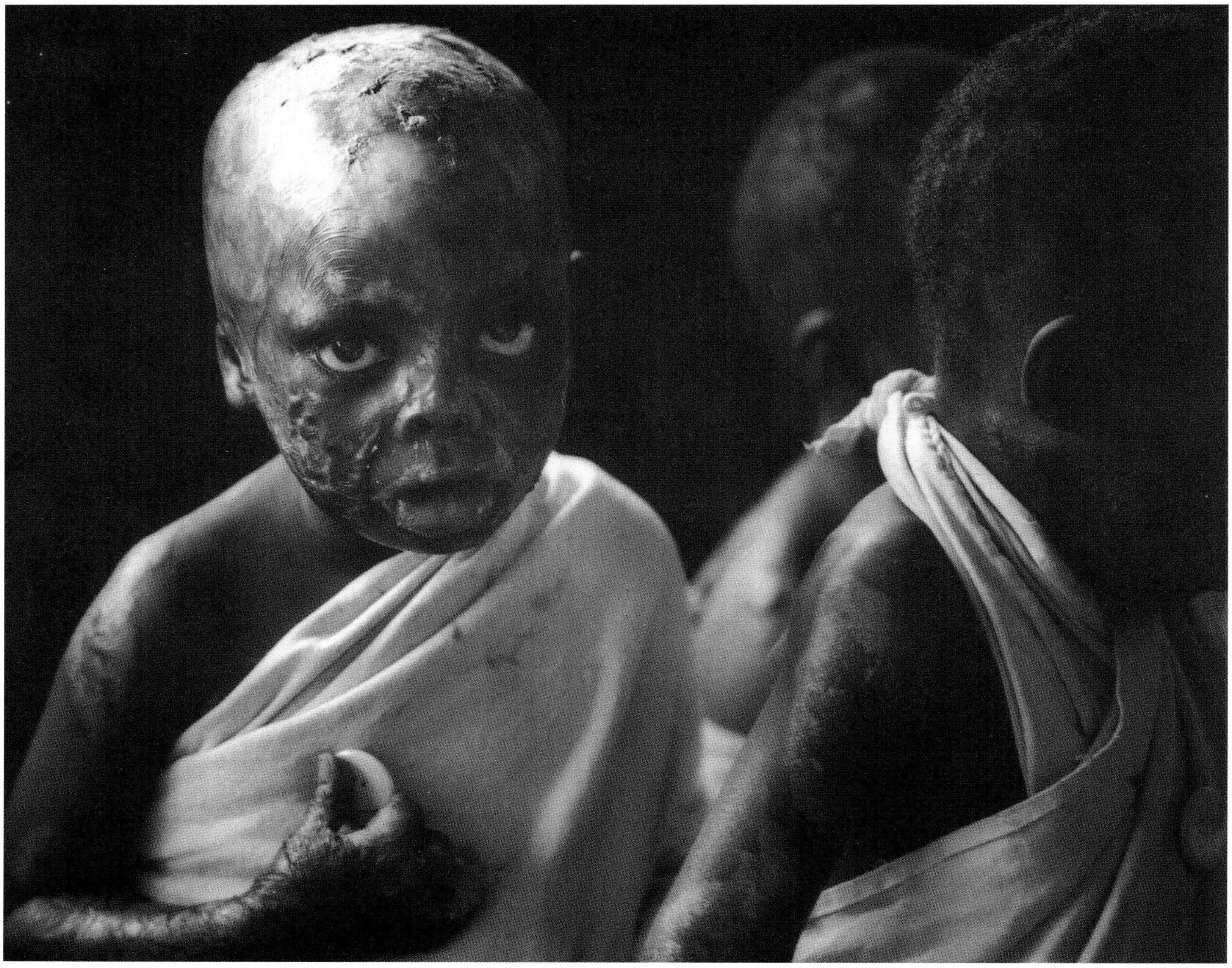

burn victims, Nairobi

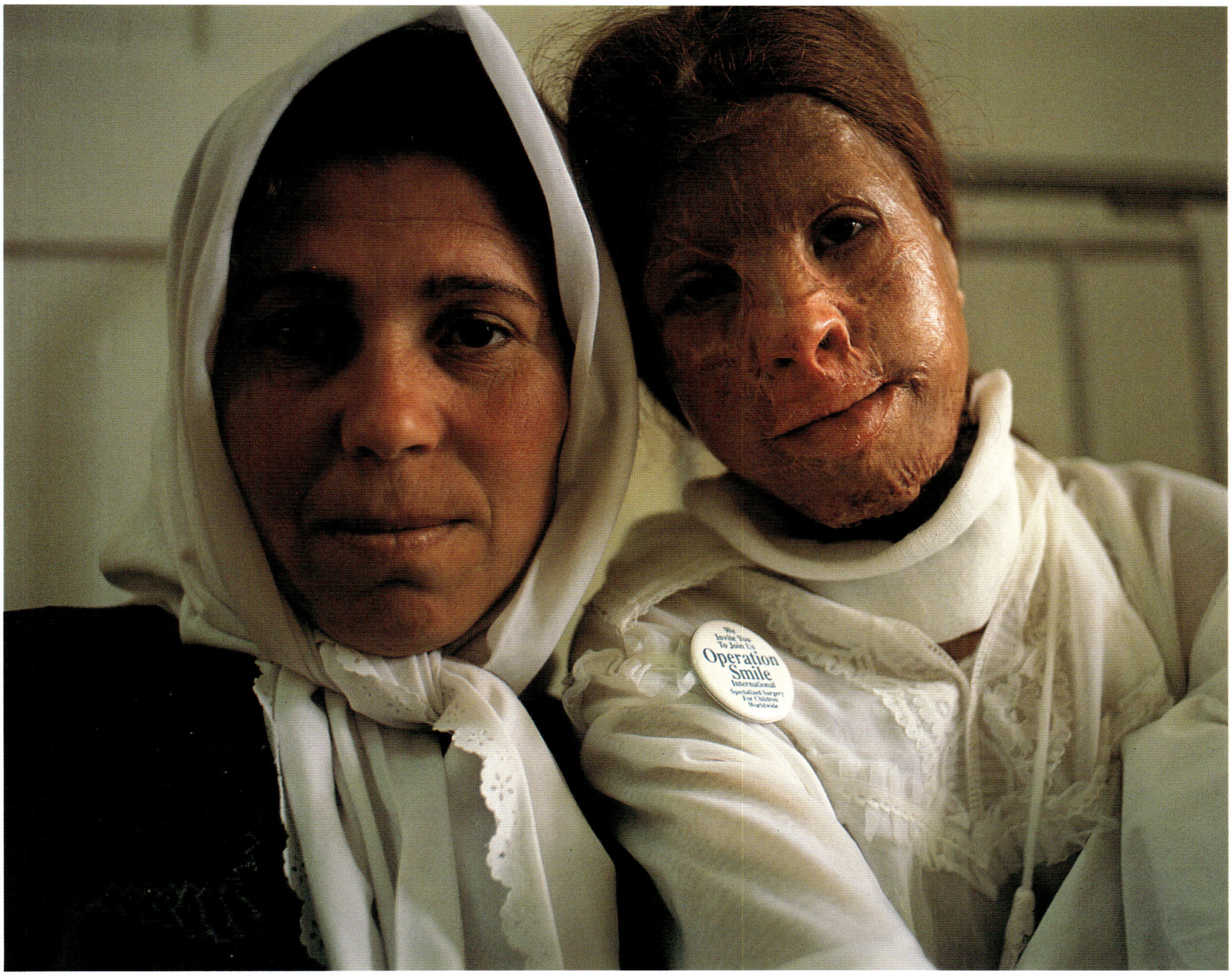

mother and daughter (burn victim), Jerusalem

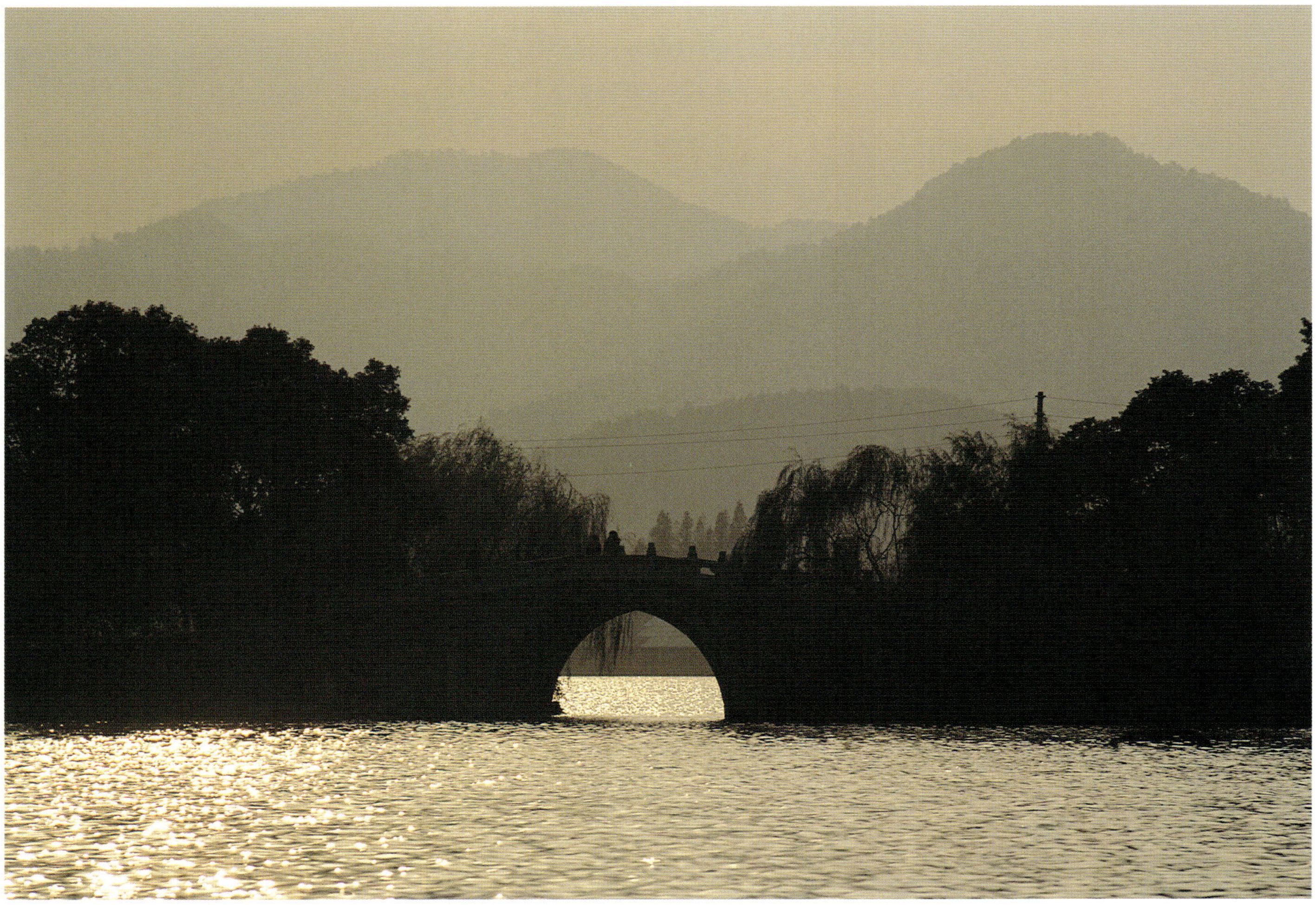

Sunset on West Lake, Hangzhou

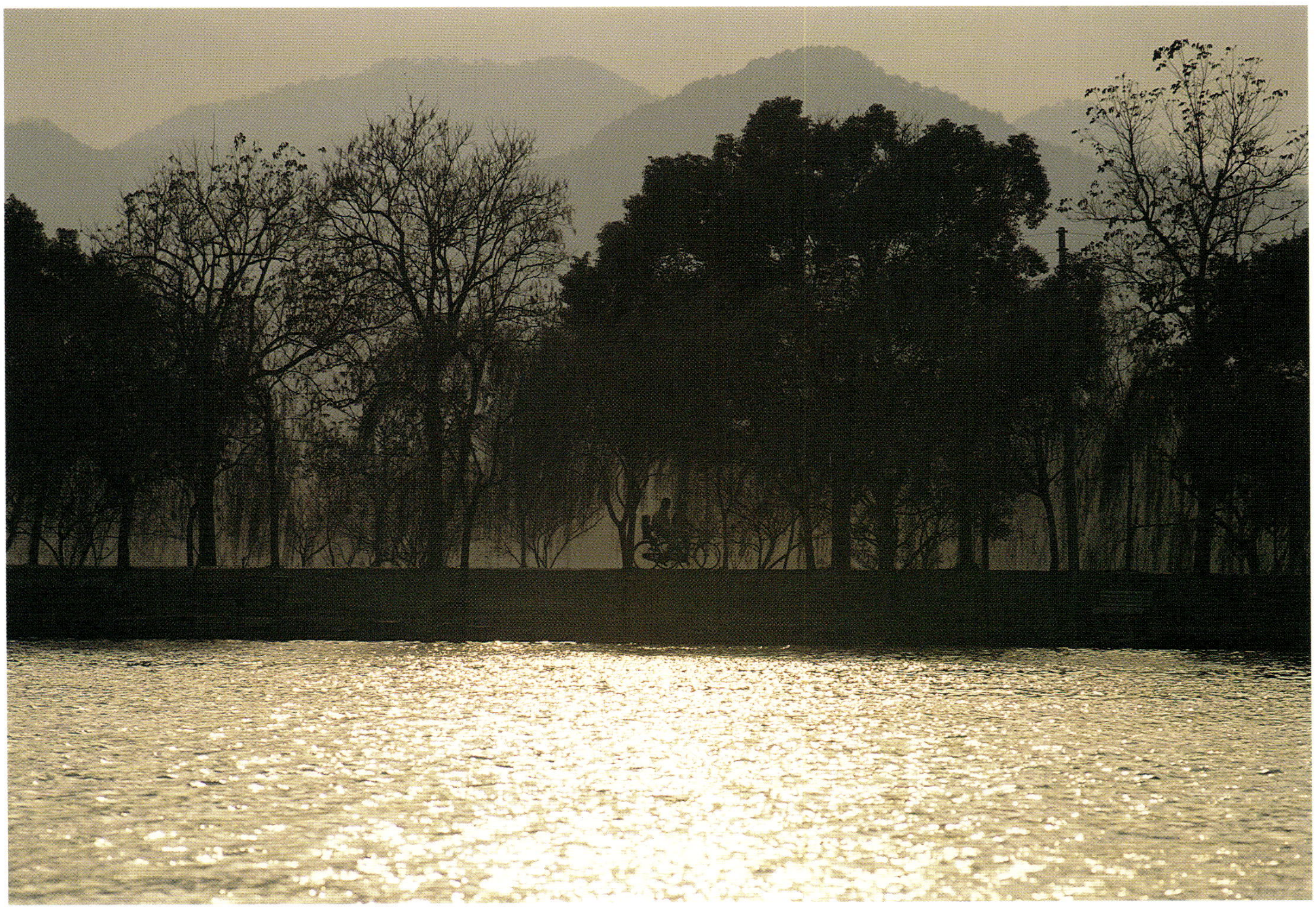

Sunset on West Lake, Hangzhou

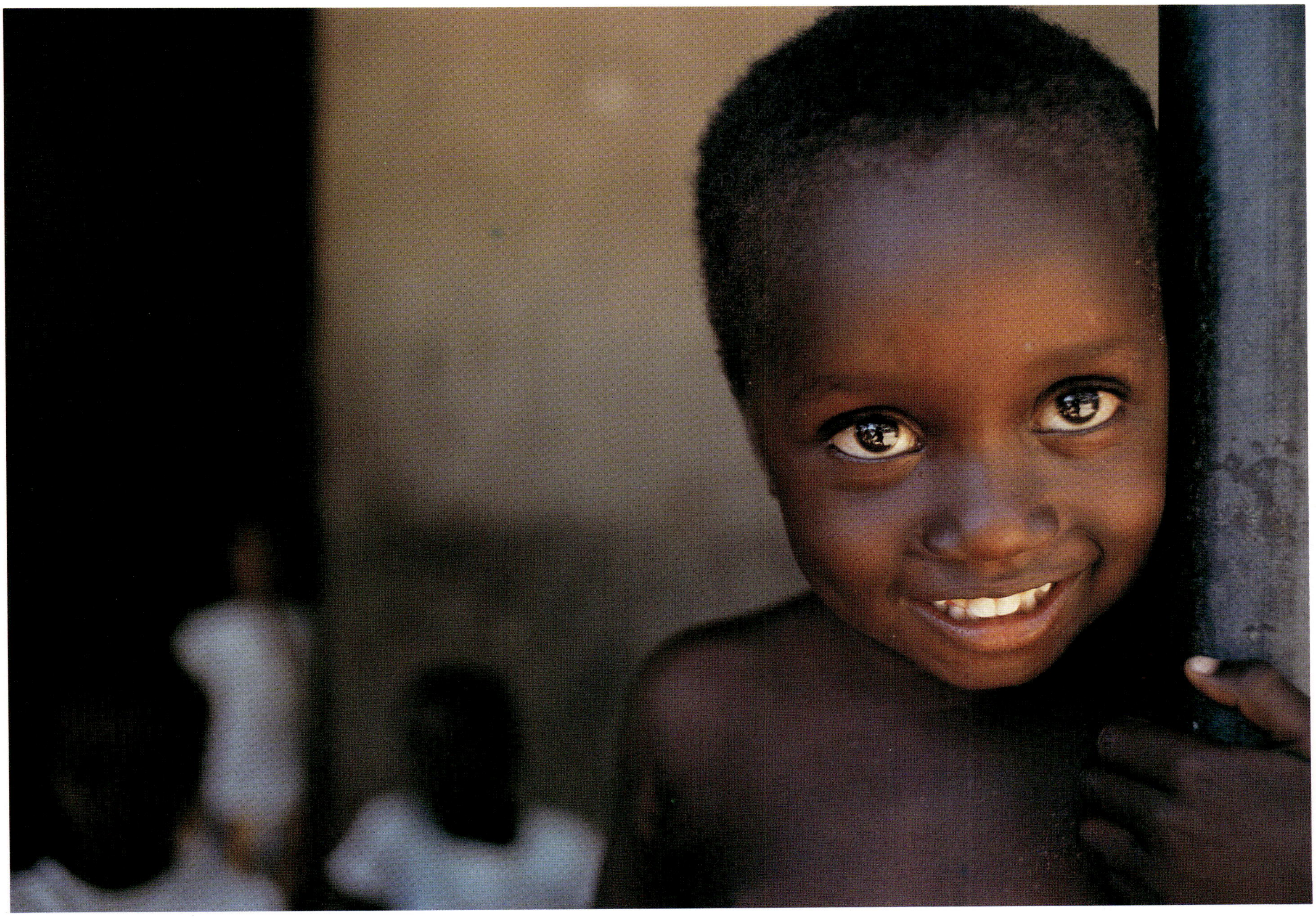

boy outside hospital, Monrovia

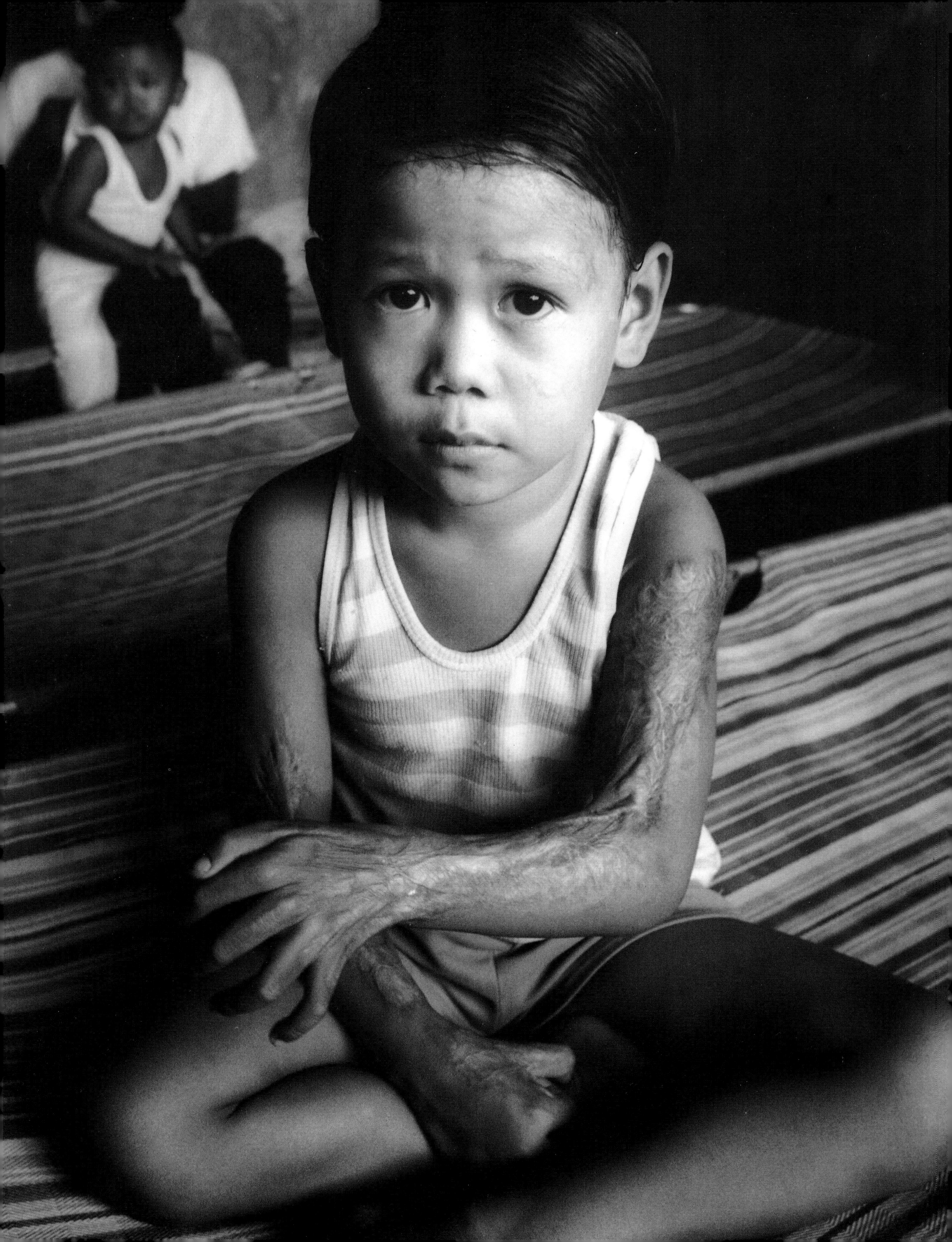

We have within our grasp the ability to change the future of a disfigured child, and by doing so, demonstrate that involvement creates change.

BILL & KATHY MAGEE
CO-FOUNDERS
OPERATION SMILE INTERNATIONAL

child with burn scars, Negros

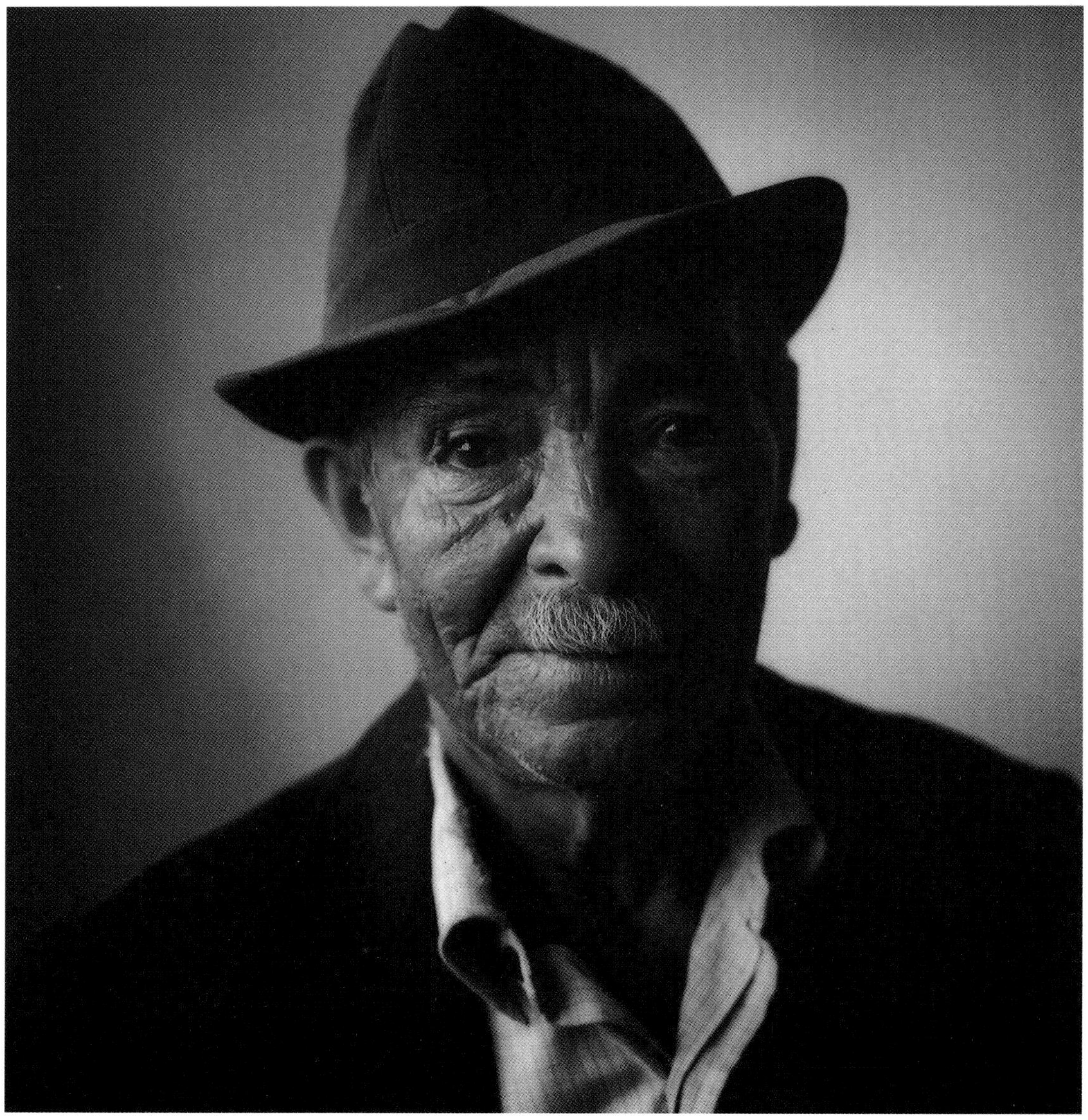

patient fathers, Manizales

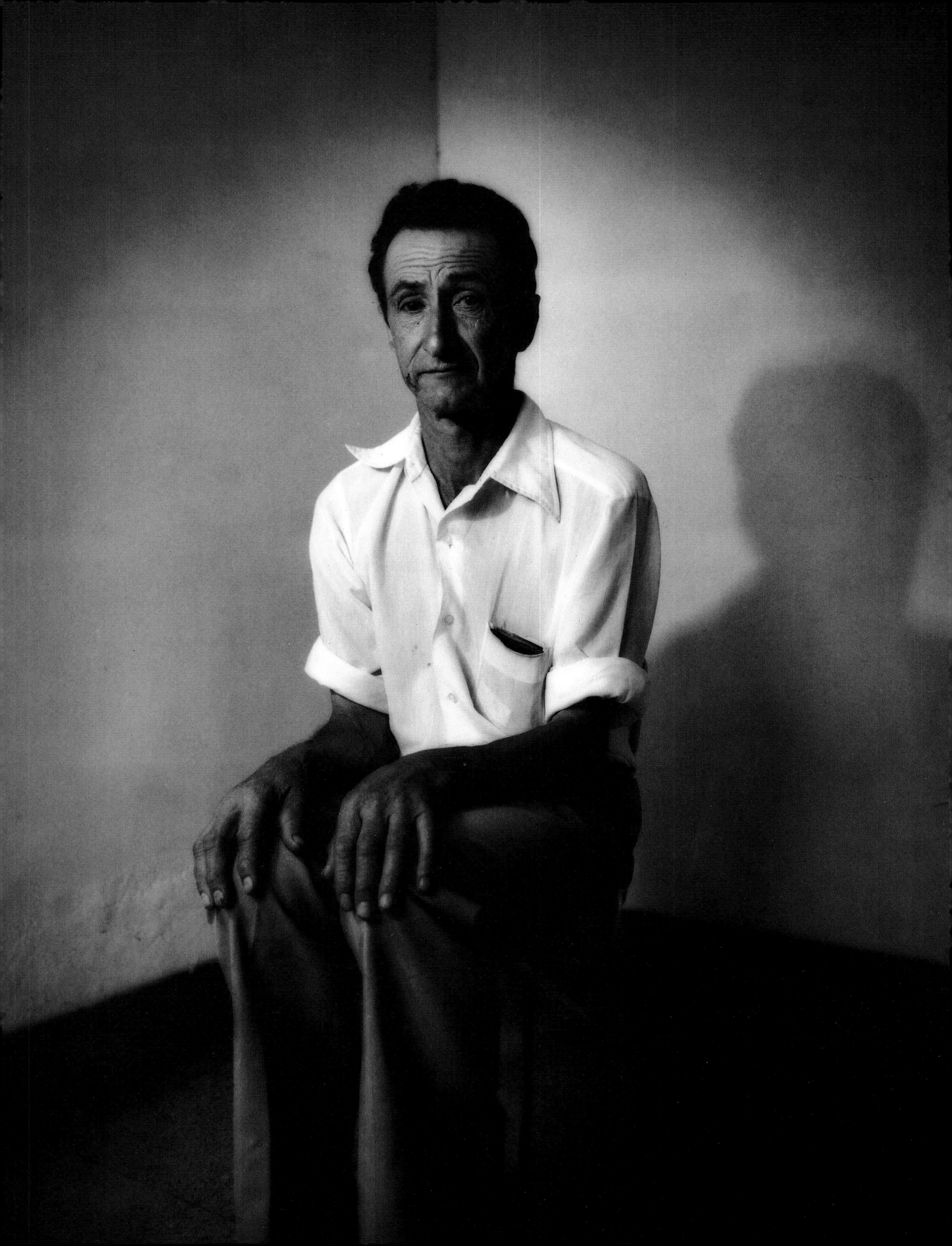

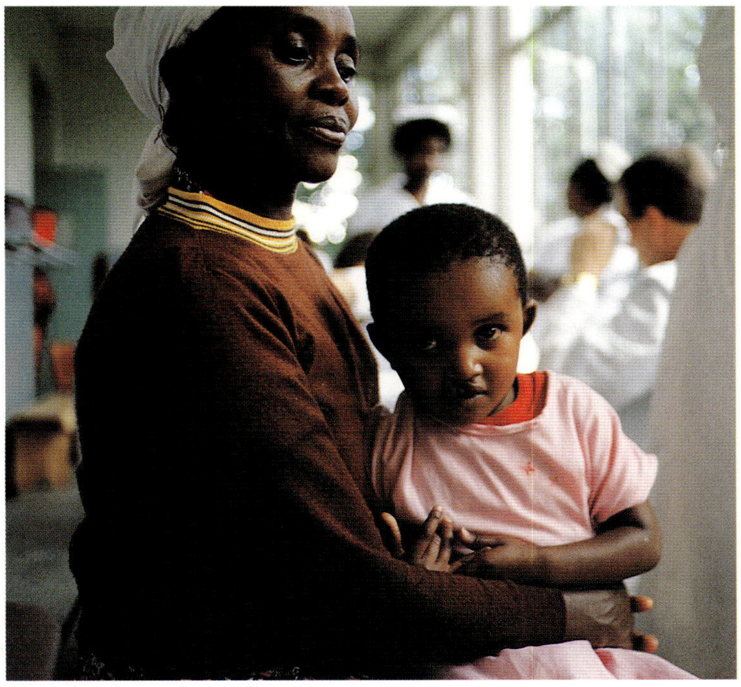

mother and son in screening, Nairobi

What started as an idea to help just a few children has grown into a mission that has transformed the lives of thousands.

BILL & KATHY MAGEE
CO-FOUNDERS
OPERATION SMILE INTERNATIONAL

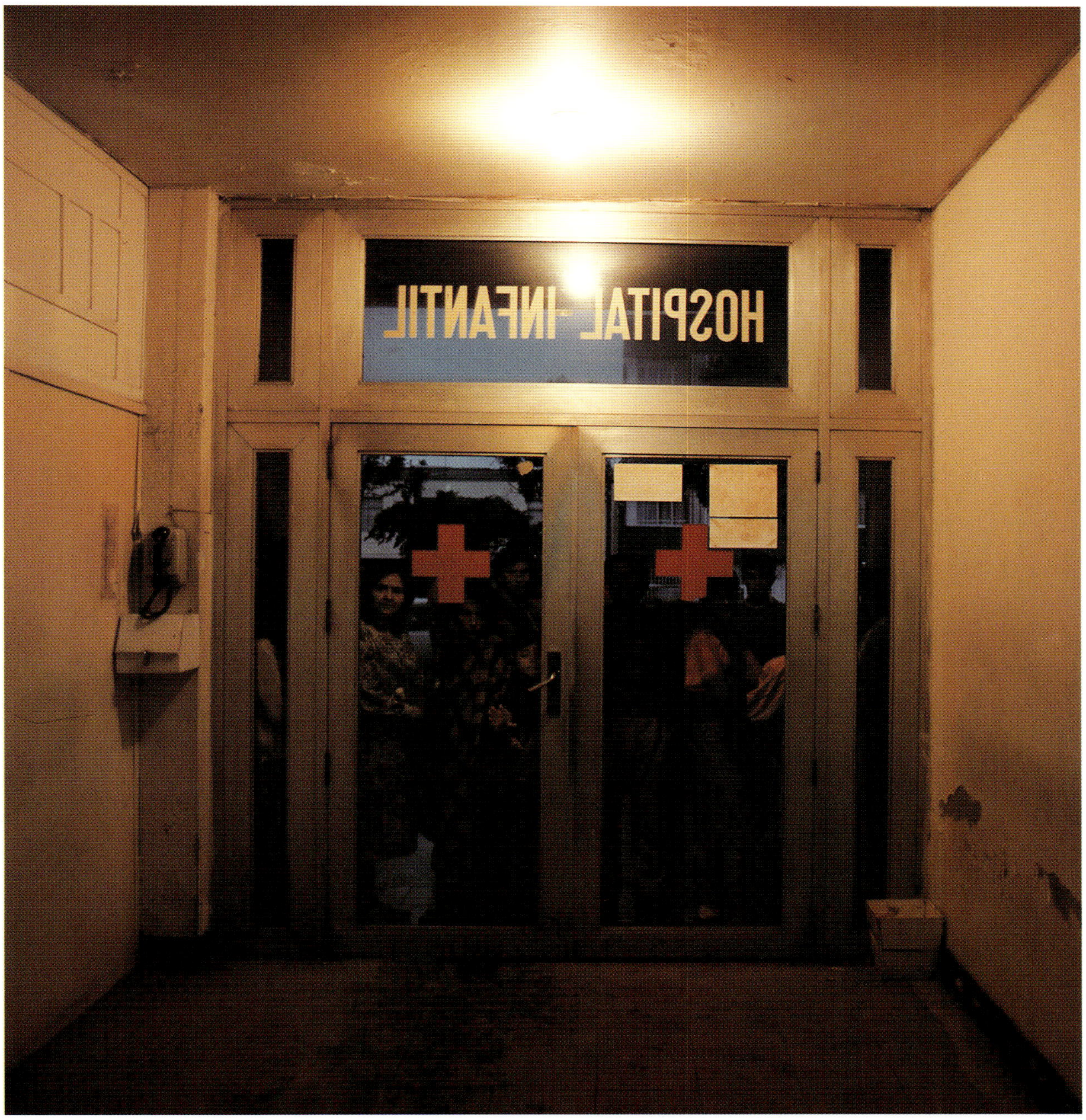

families wait outside hospital, Manizales
(previous spread) sunset in the National Park, Nairobi

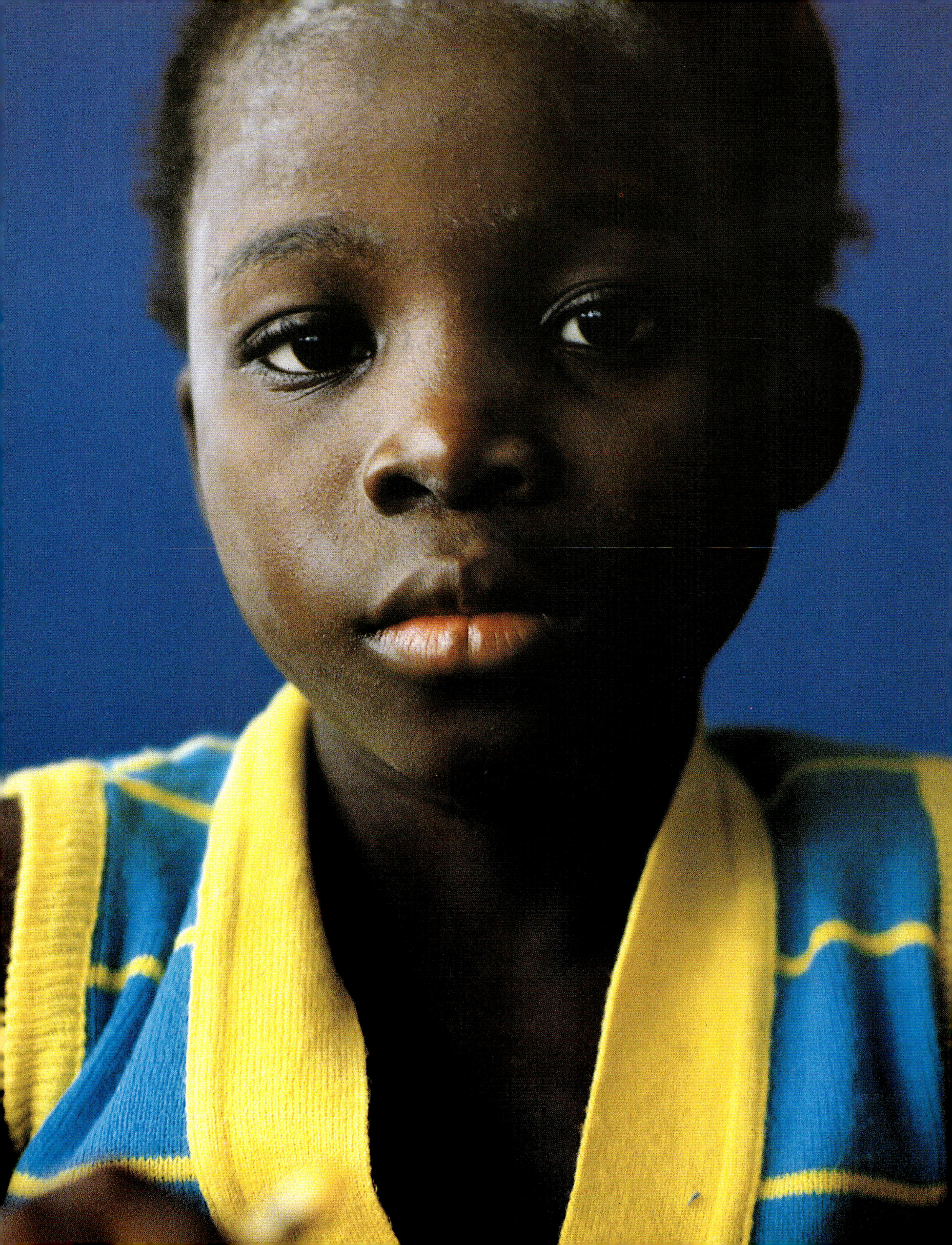

patient on children's ward, Monrovia

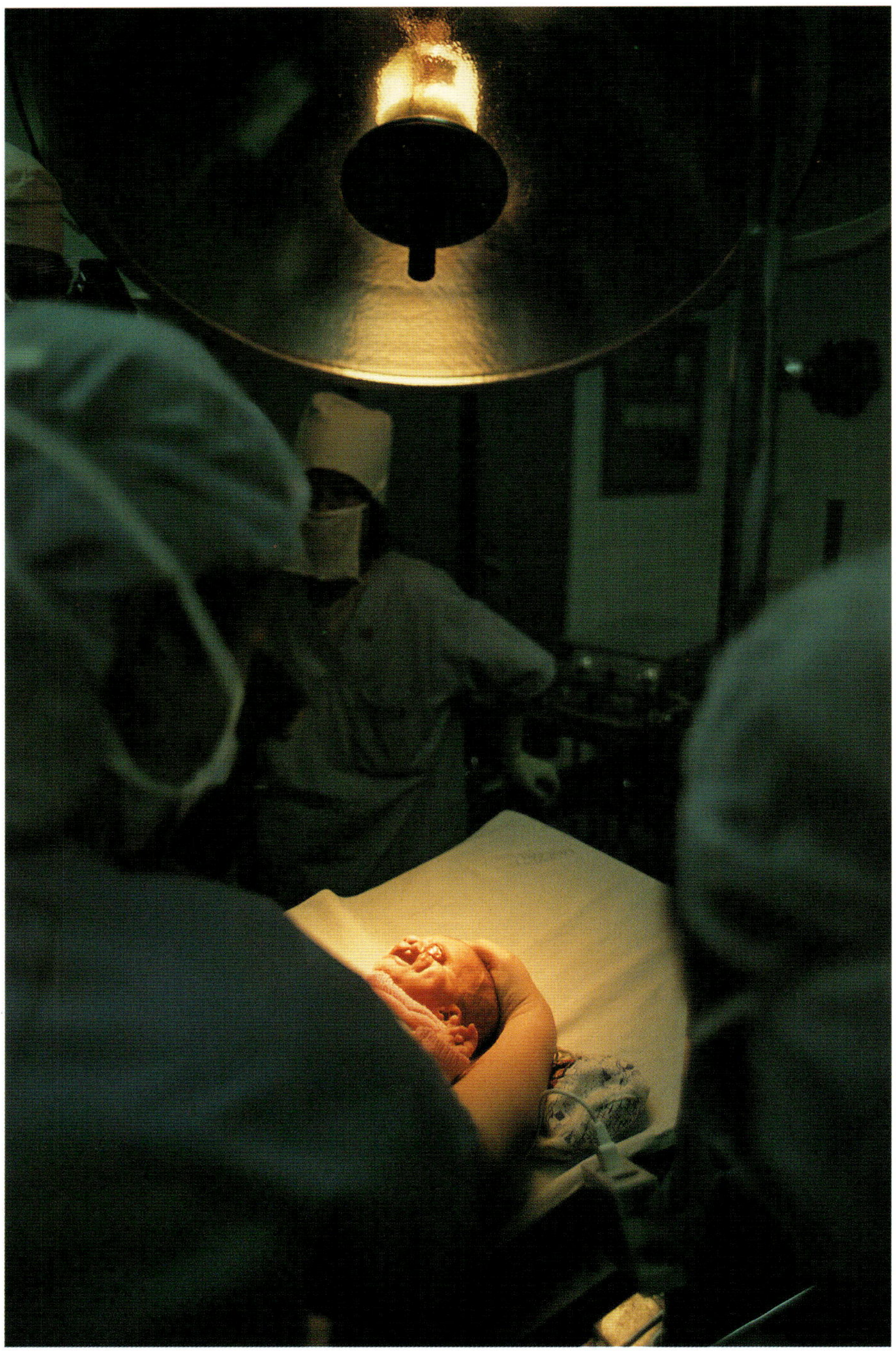

child in surgery, Hanoi
lip and palate surgery, Panama City (photograph by Taro Yamasaki)

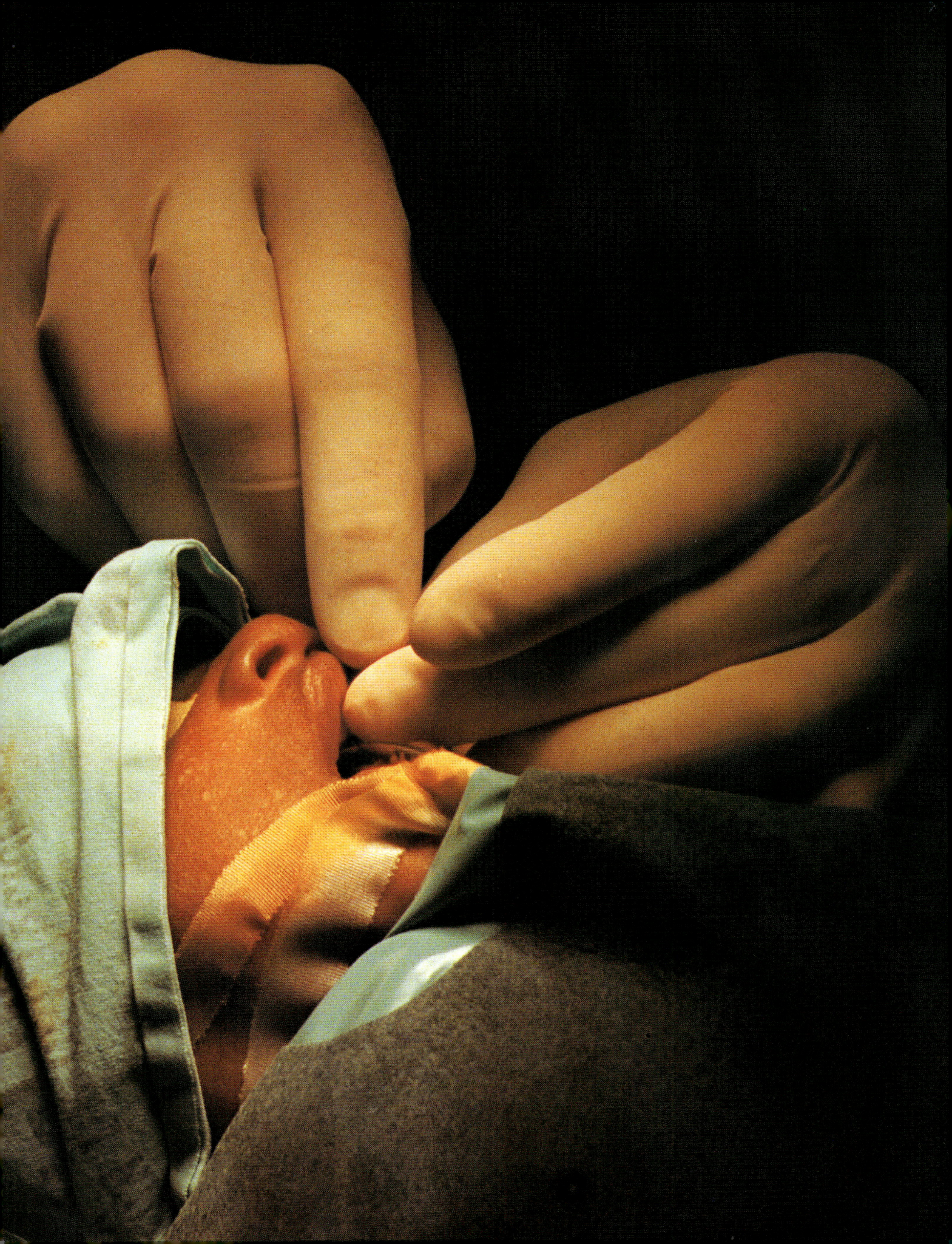

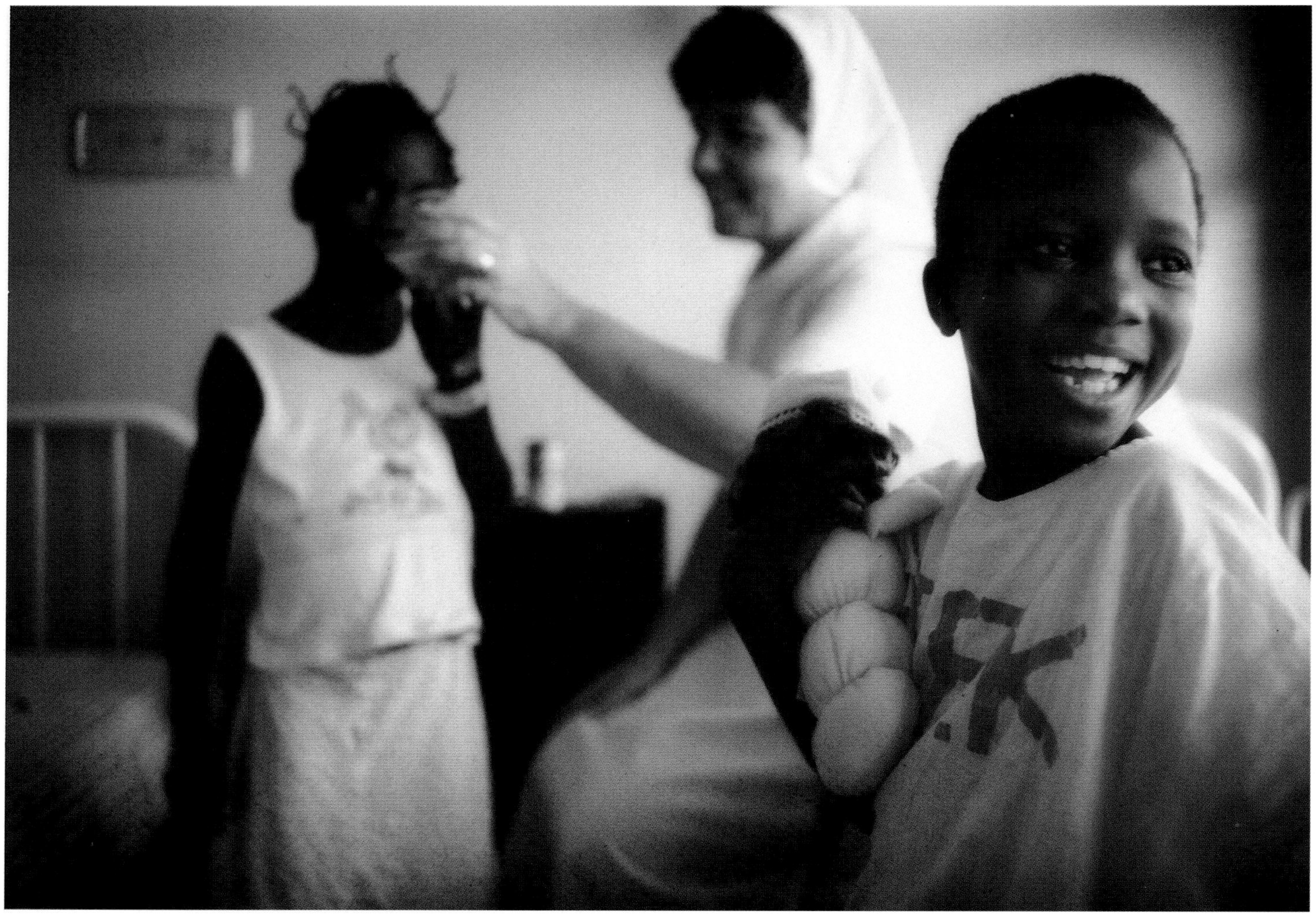

children await treatment, Monrovia

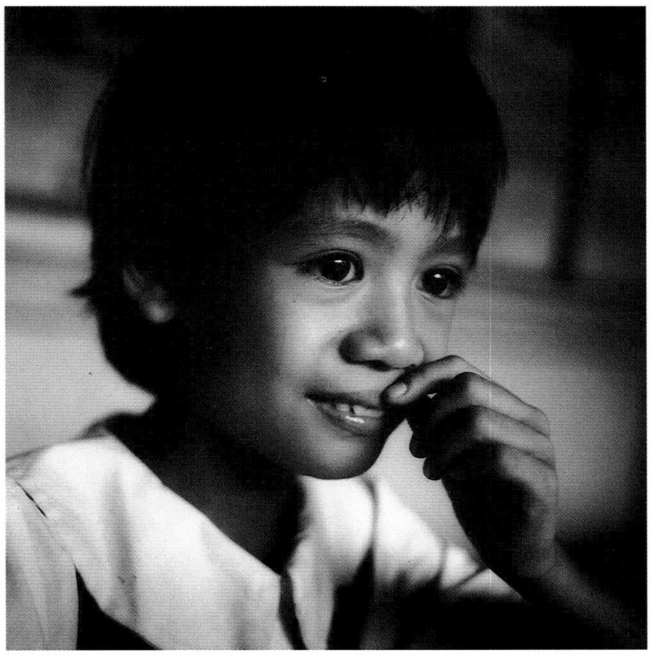

schoolgirl, Negros

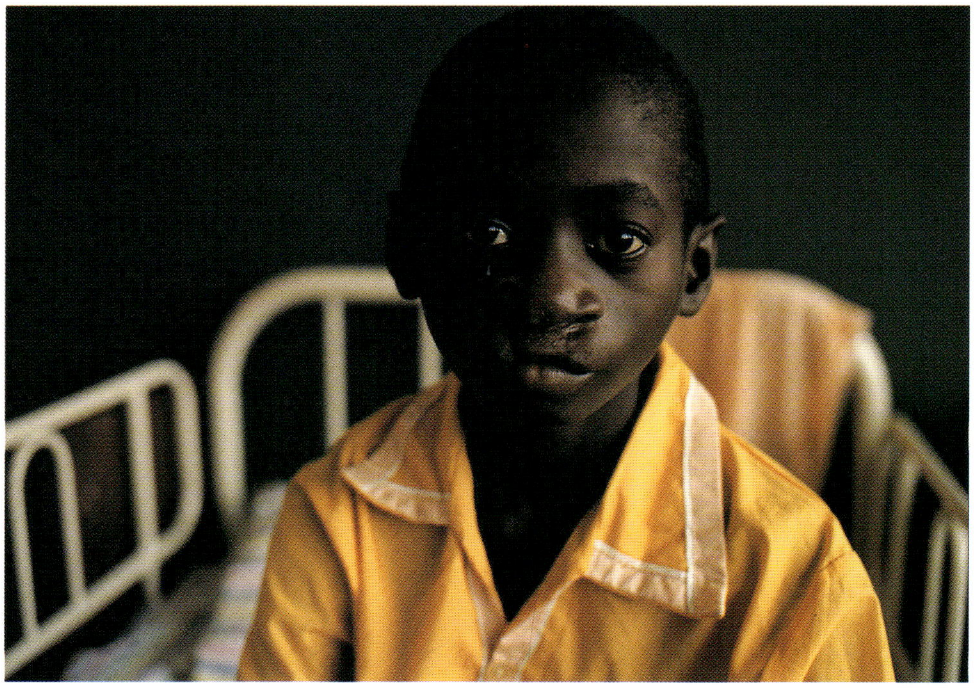

patient in pre-op, Monrovia

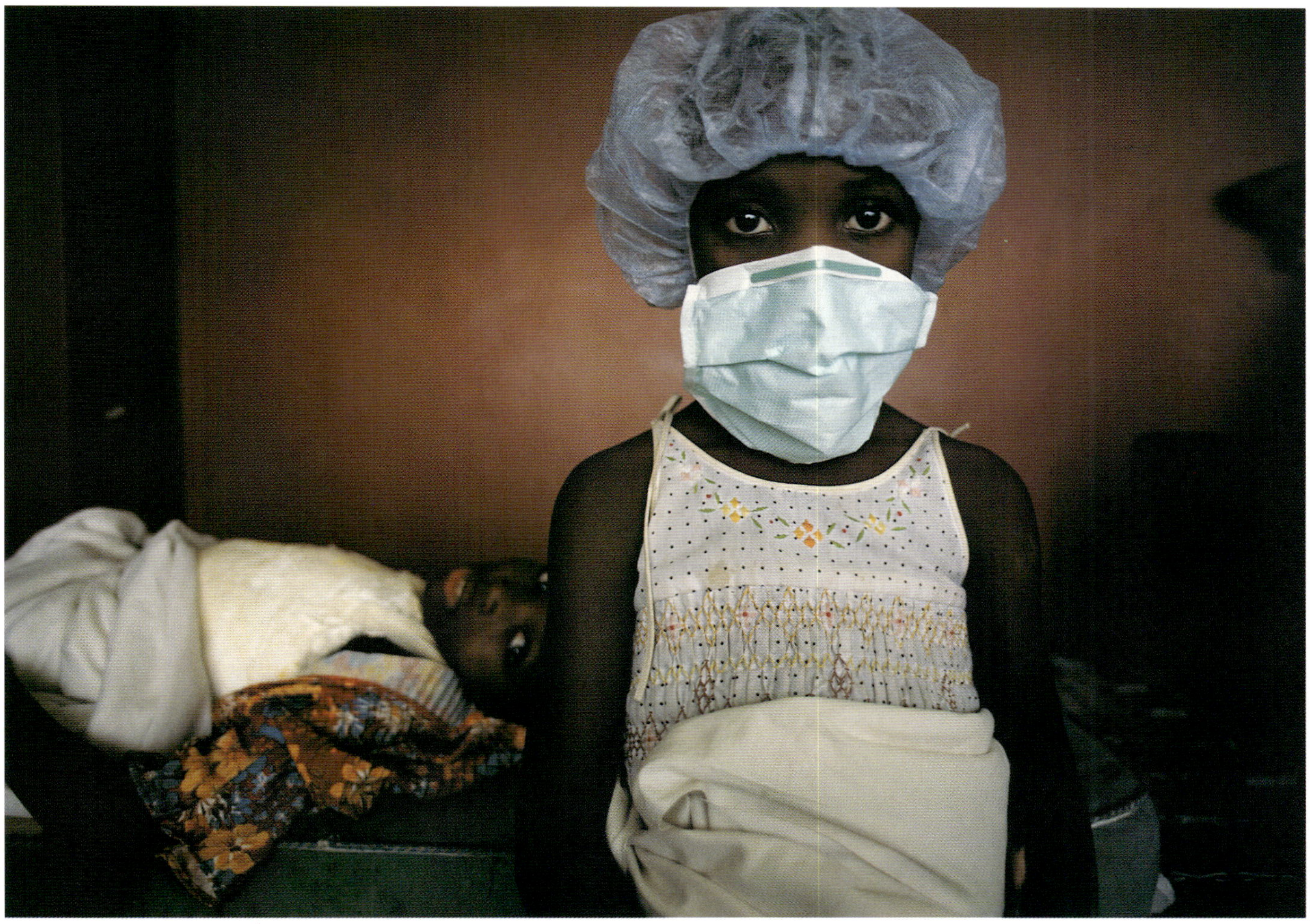

children in pre-op, Monrovia

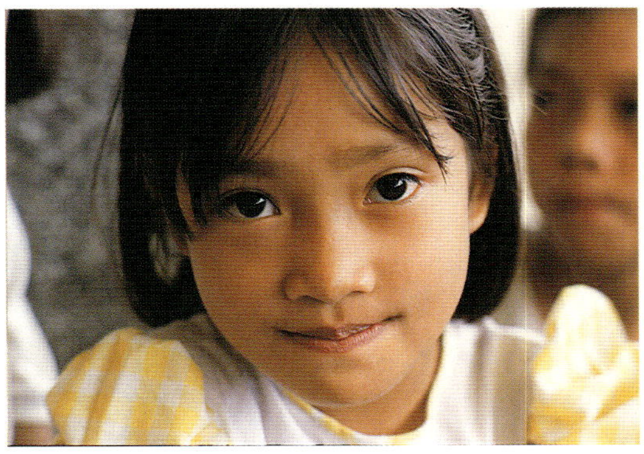

I have learned much about gifts and giving,
and the love that goes into each.

This is Operation Smile's gift to each one of us.

NORMAN THOMAS SCOTT, MD
OSI MEDICAL VOLUNTEER

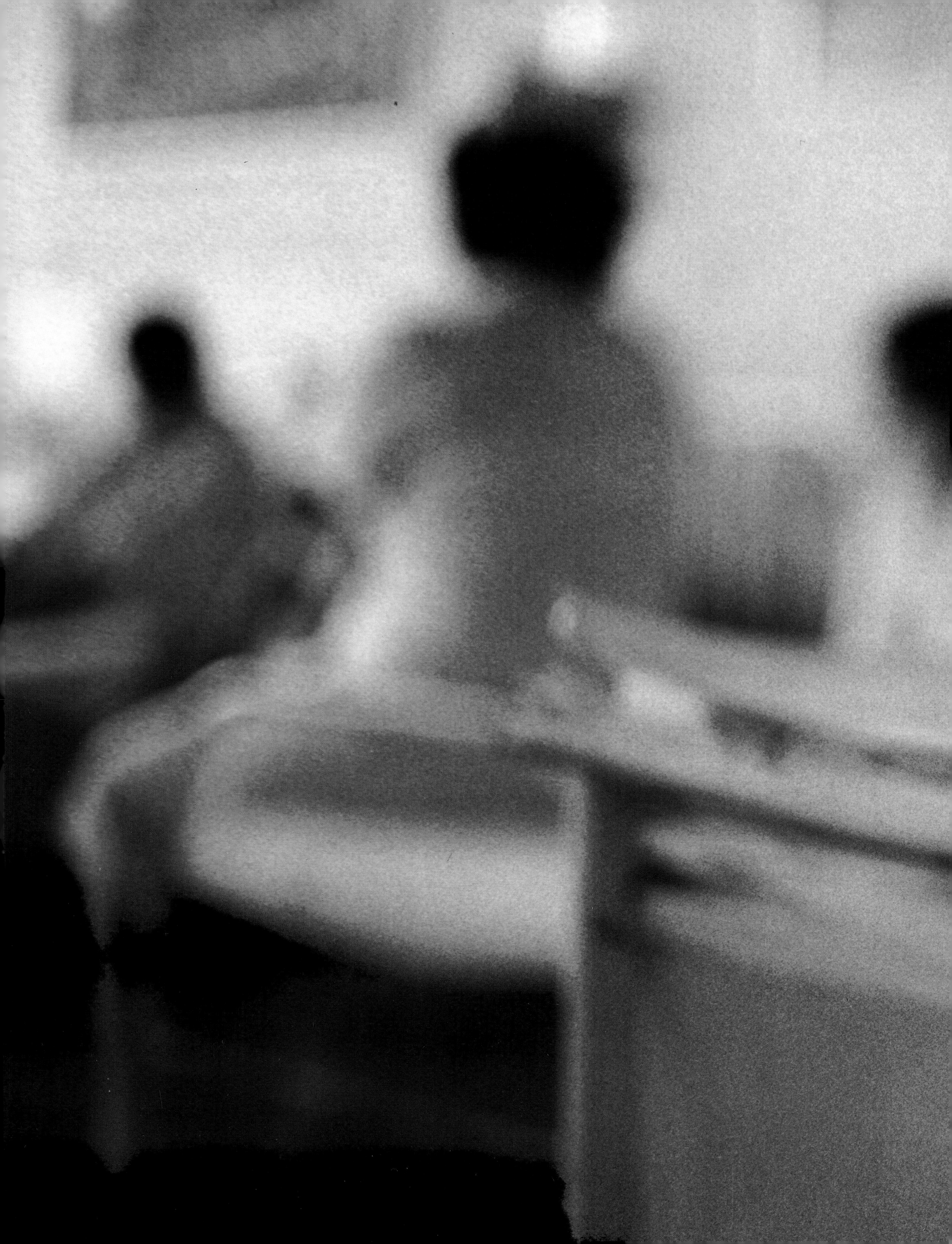

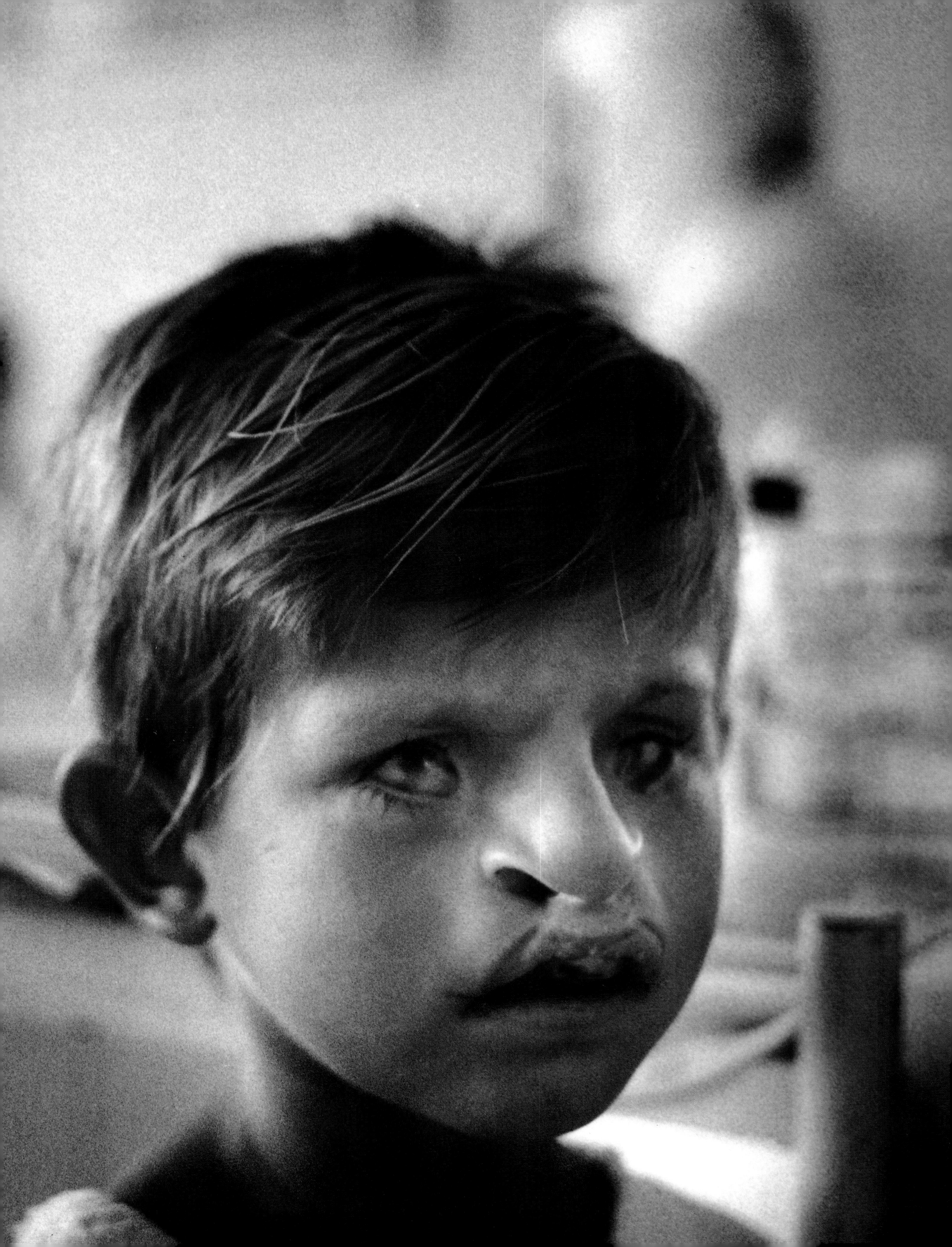

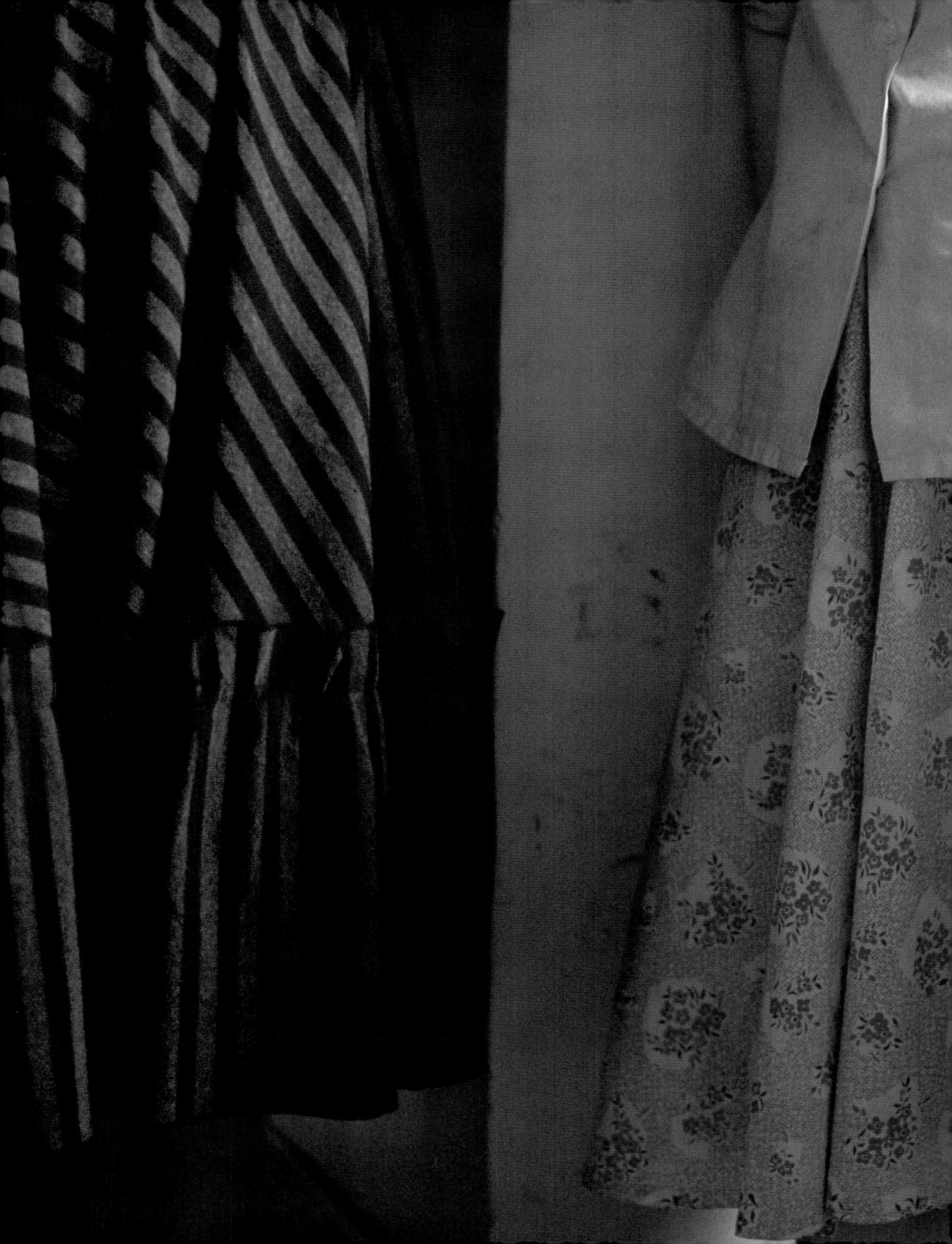

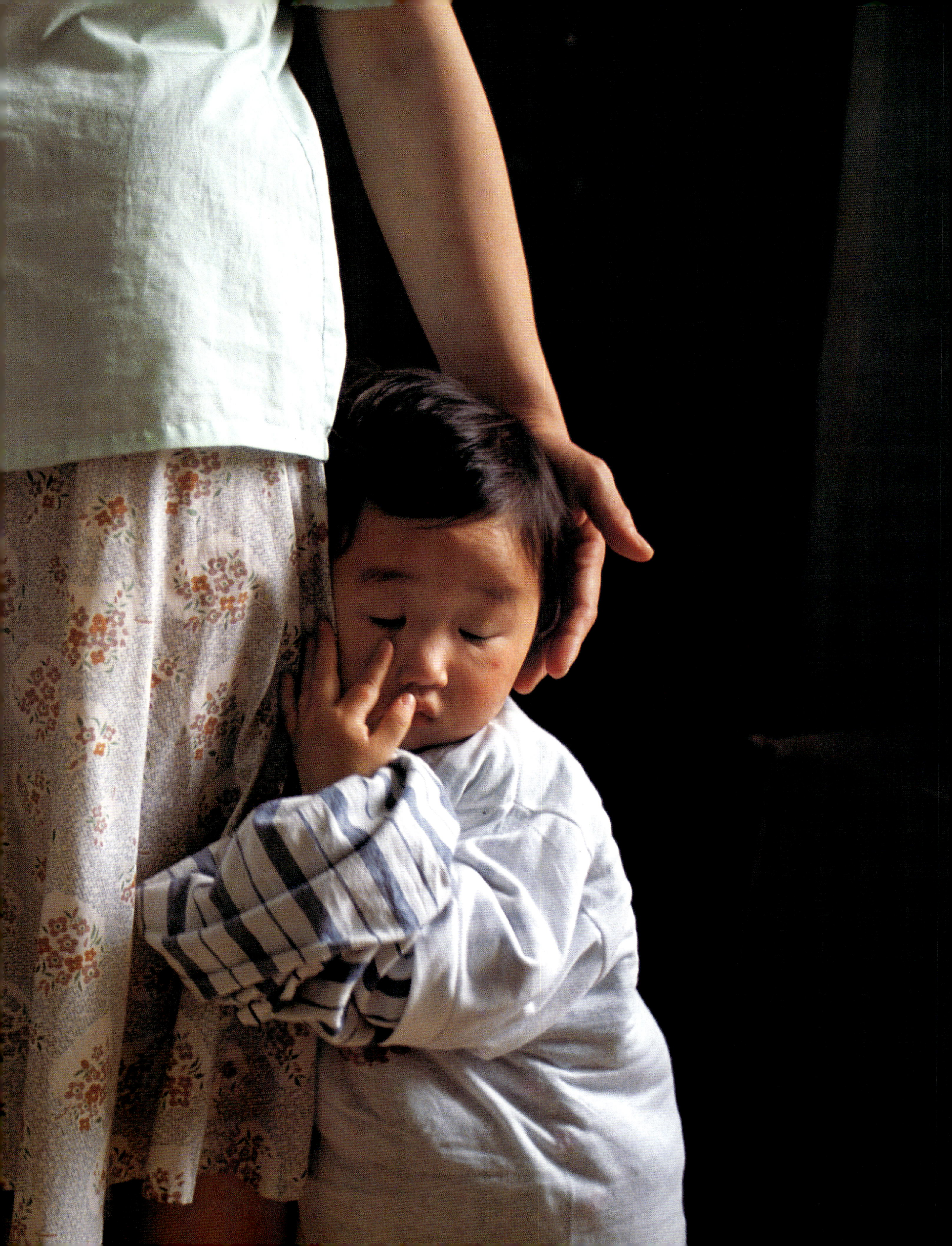

(previous spreads)
boy on pre-op ward, Manizales
mother and child, Hangzhou

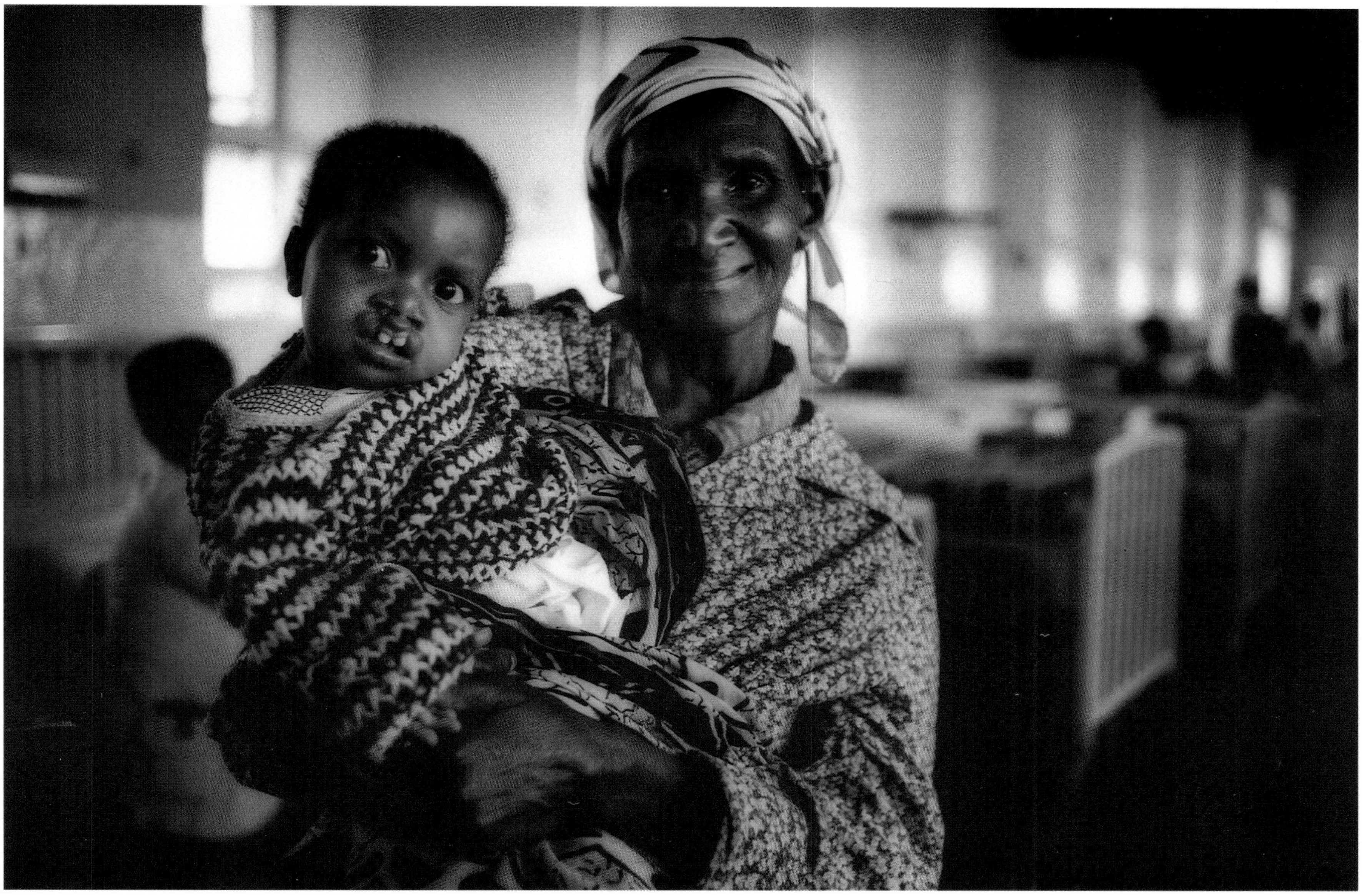

mother and child, Nairobi

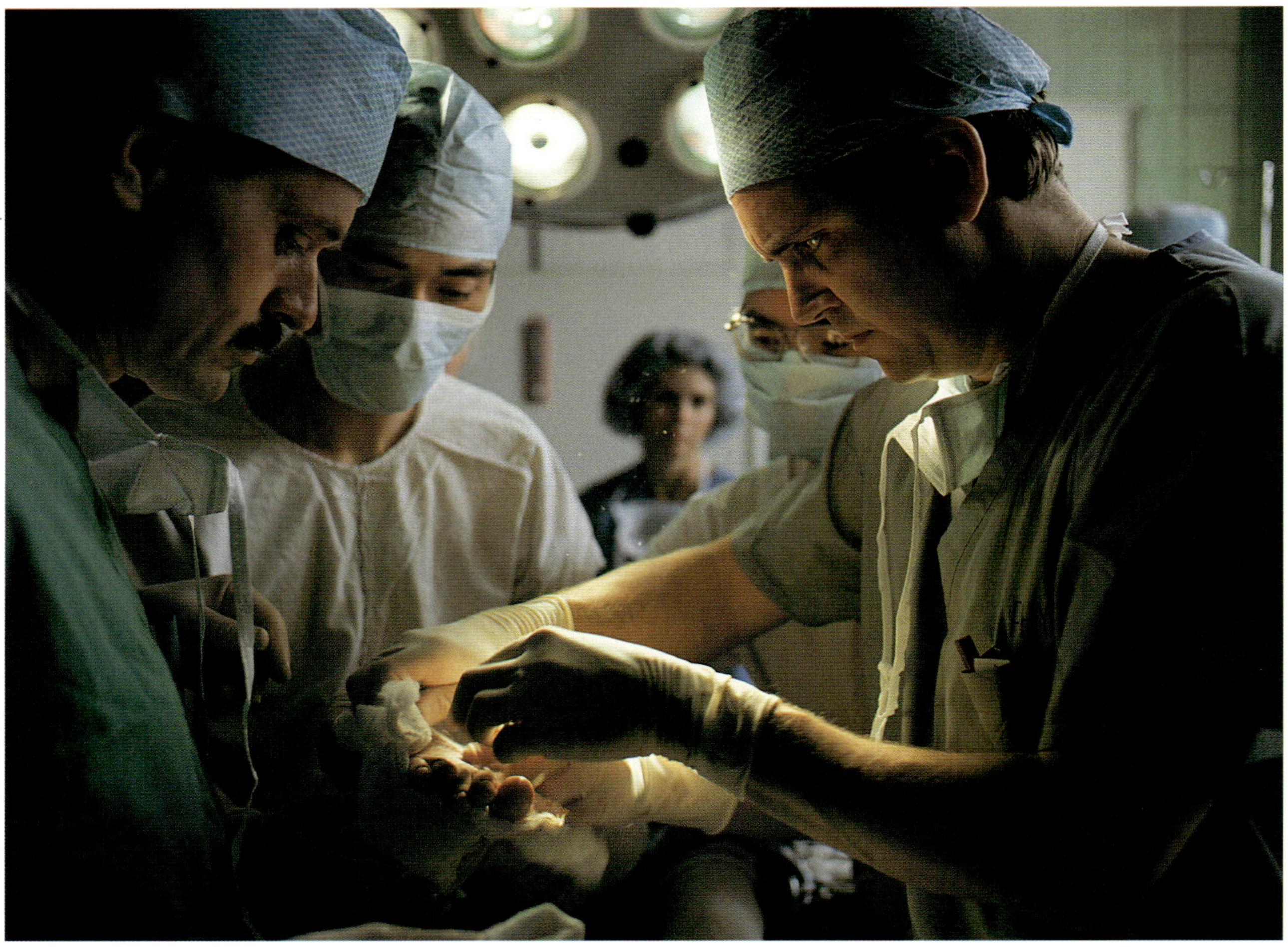

casting, Hangzhou

In our humanitarian pursuits, we have three encompassing possessions: our time, our talent, and our treasure. Our time, of course, we cannot keep. Only that which we give to others is not lost. We also cannot keep our talent. We must use it or we lose it. Our treasure, at last, is not permanent either. Most of us have lived long enough to know that we really only keep that which we give away.

AUTHOR UNKNOWN

patient with mother, Hangzhou

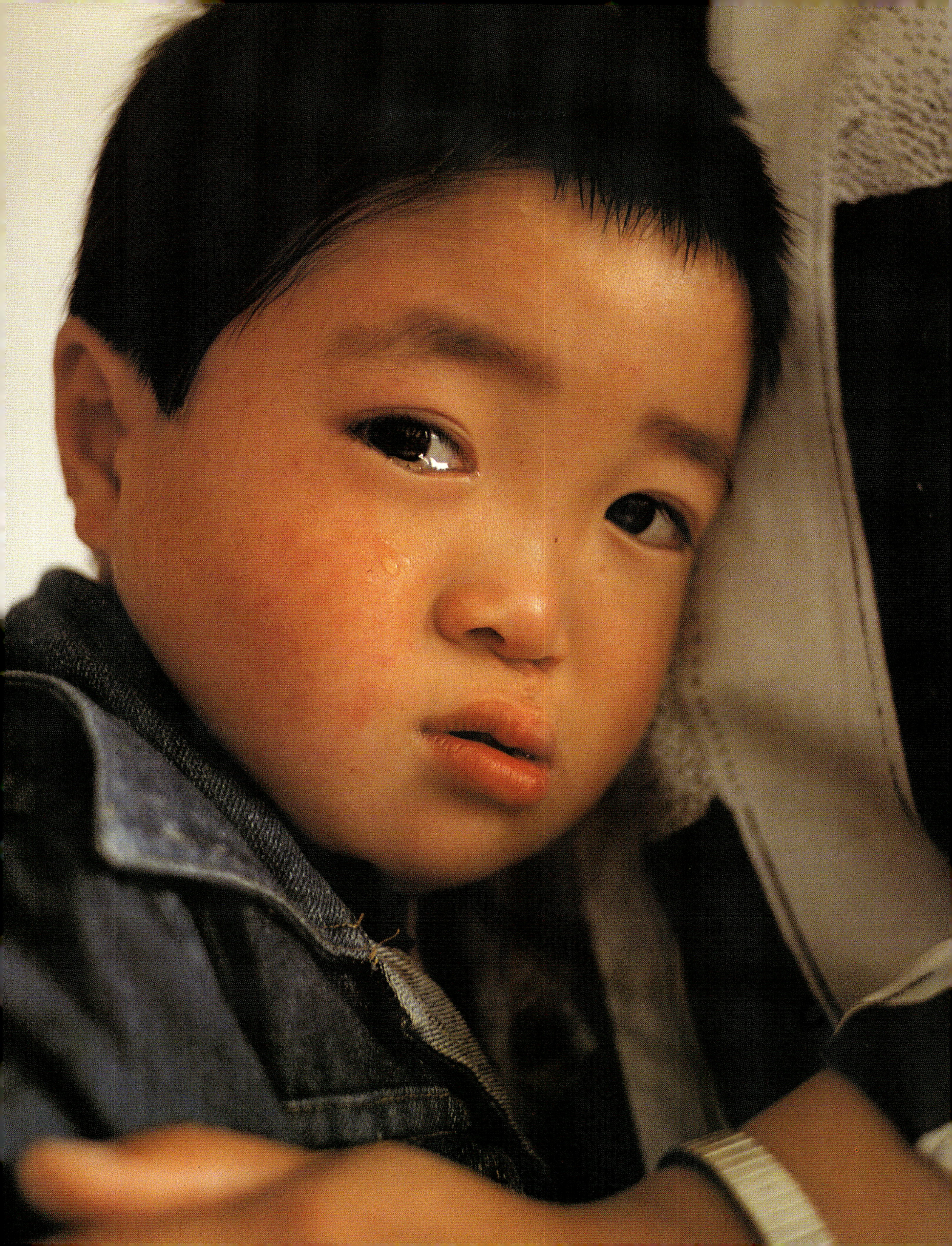

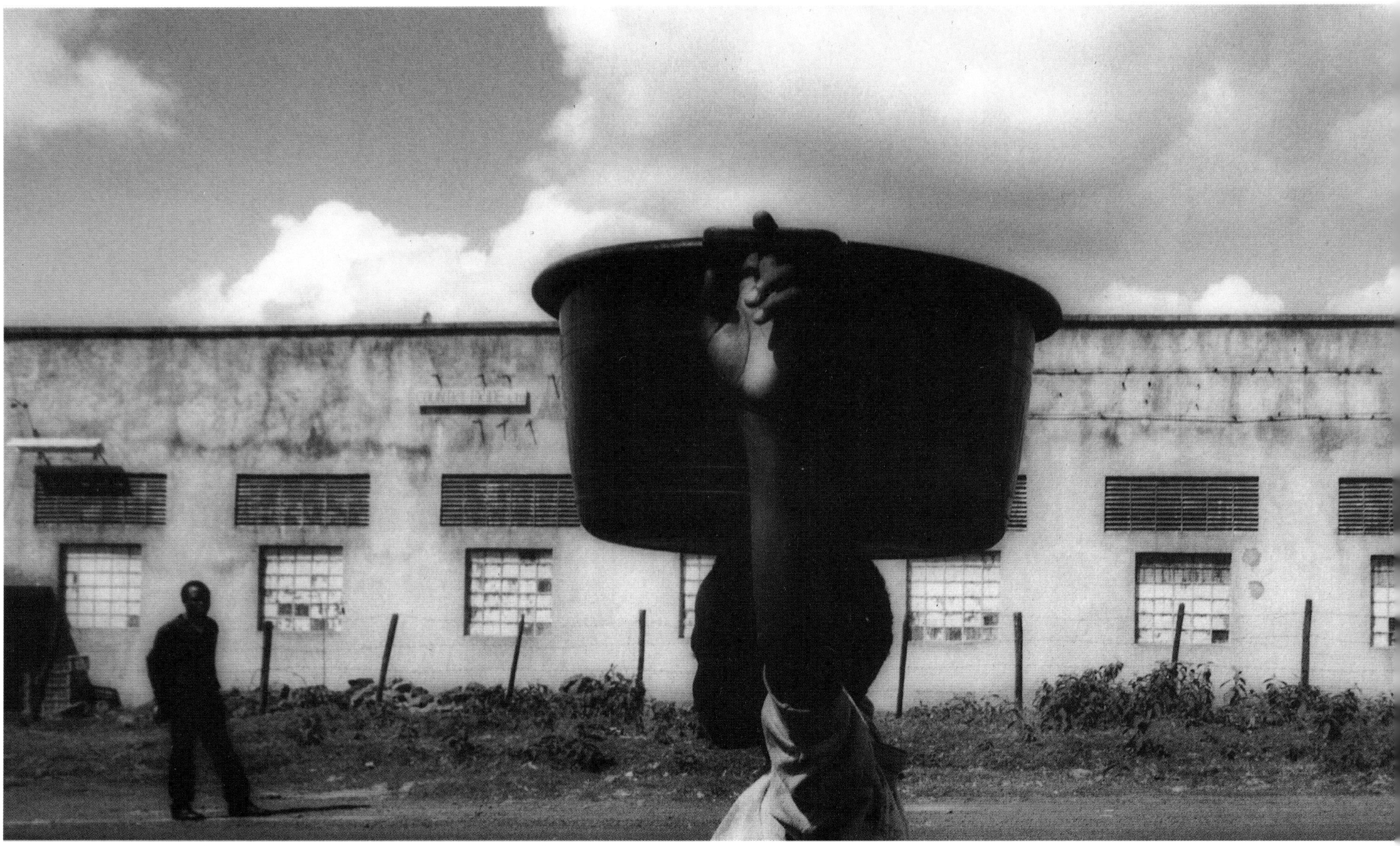

a boy and a man, Nairobi

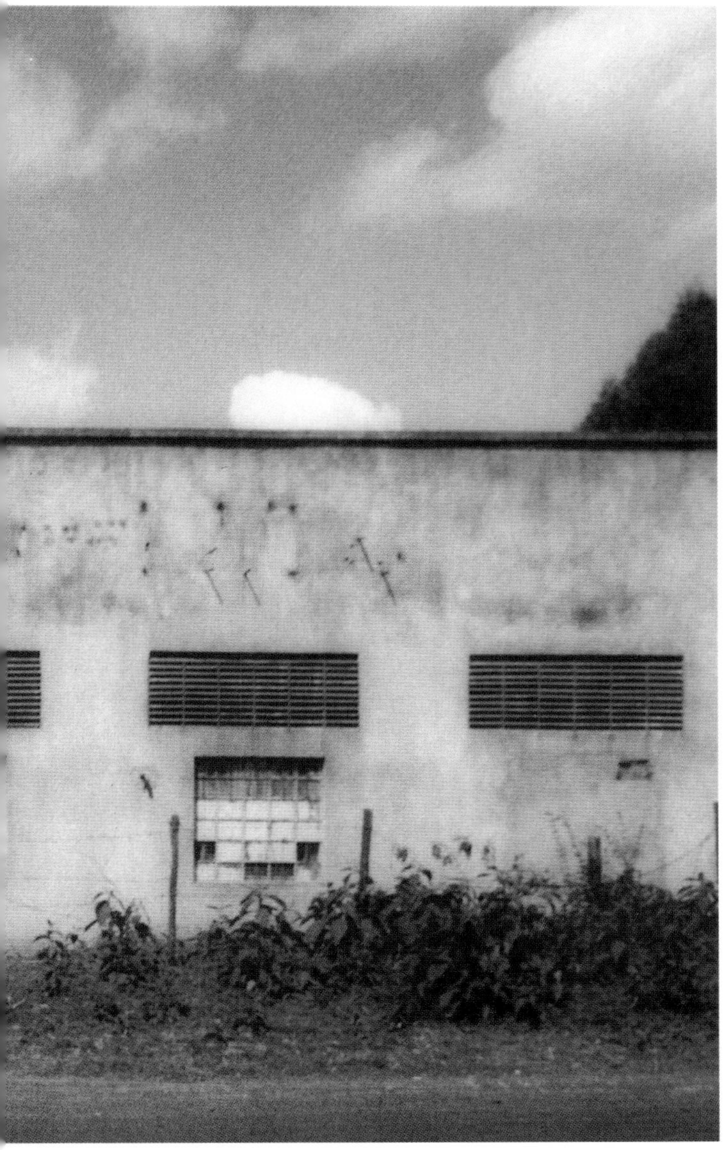

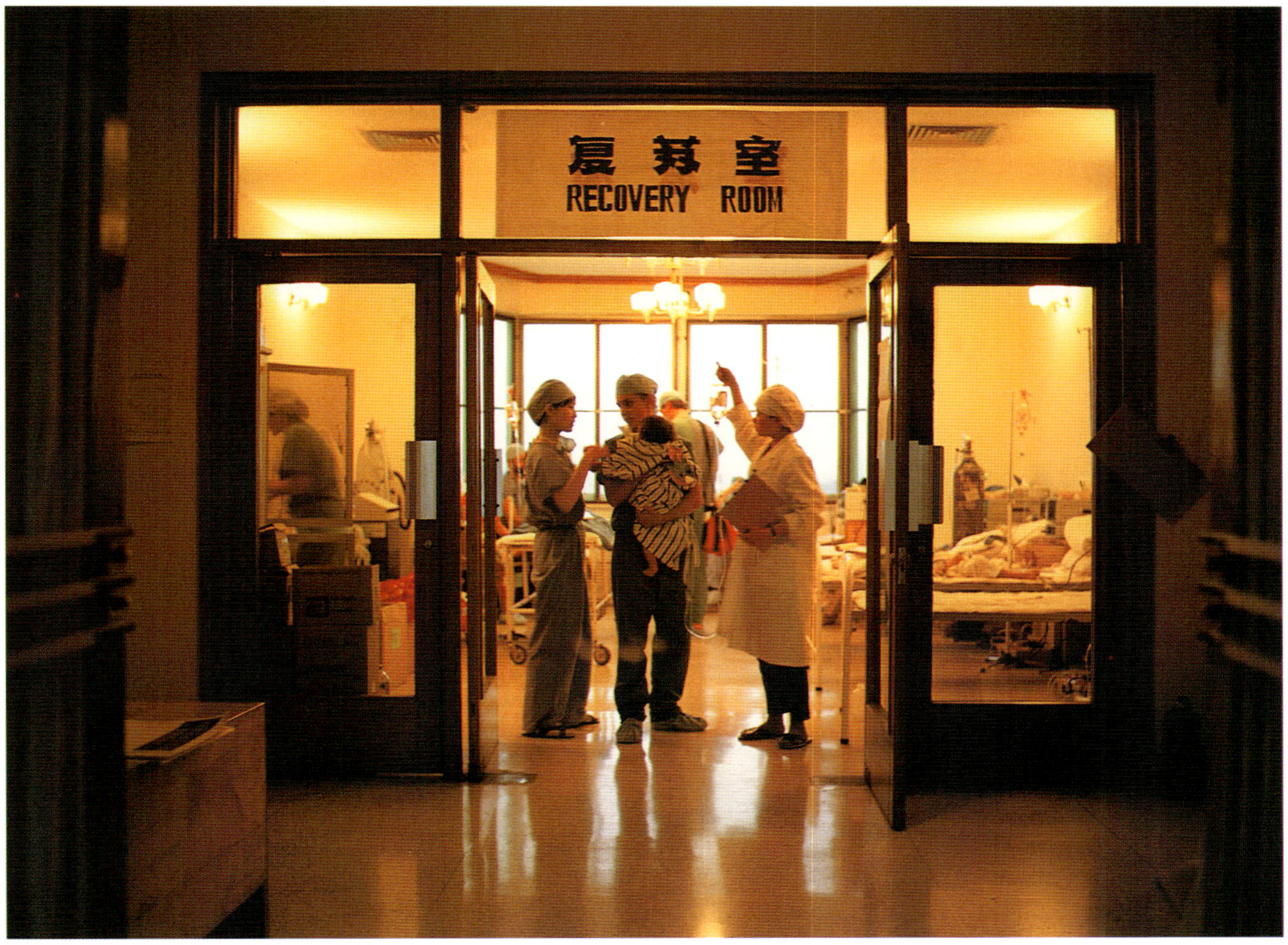

evening in the recovery room, Hangzhou

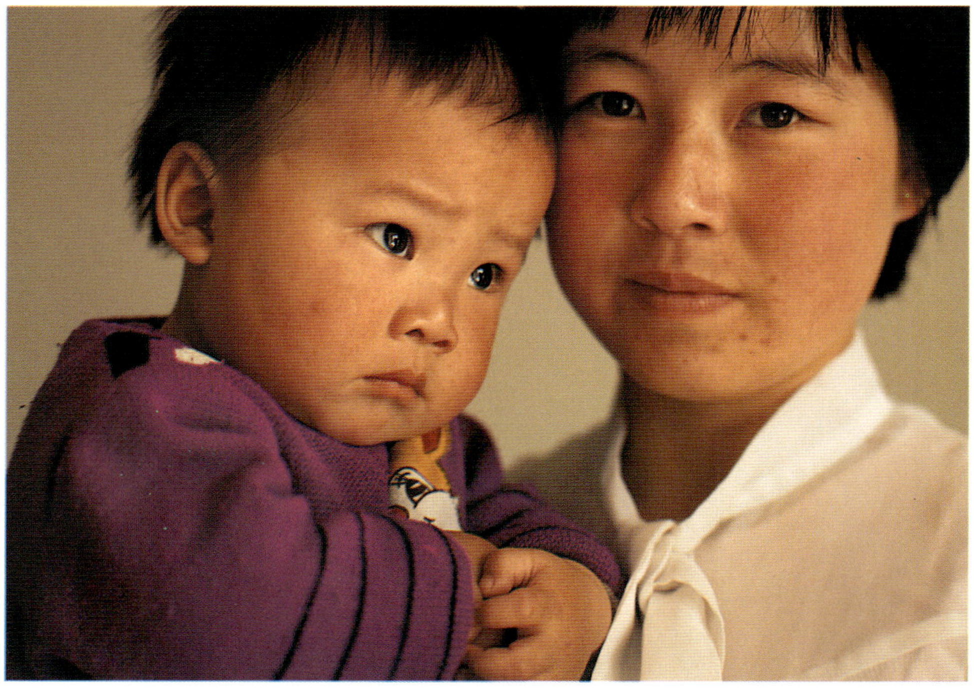

mother and child, Hangzhou

Operation Smile represents such a hopeful aspect of medicine.
A smile is the most hopeful thing you can give,
it revolutionizes both the child's and parent's lives.
When you see the parents weeping for joy
when their child comes out of surgery,
it's the most wonderful thing to experience.

KATHY MILLER
OSI VOLUNTEER

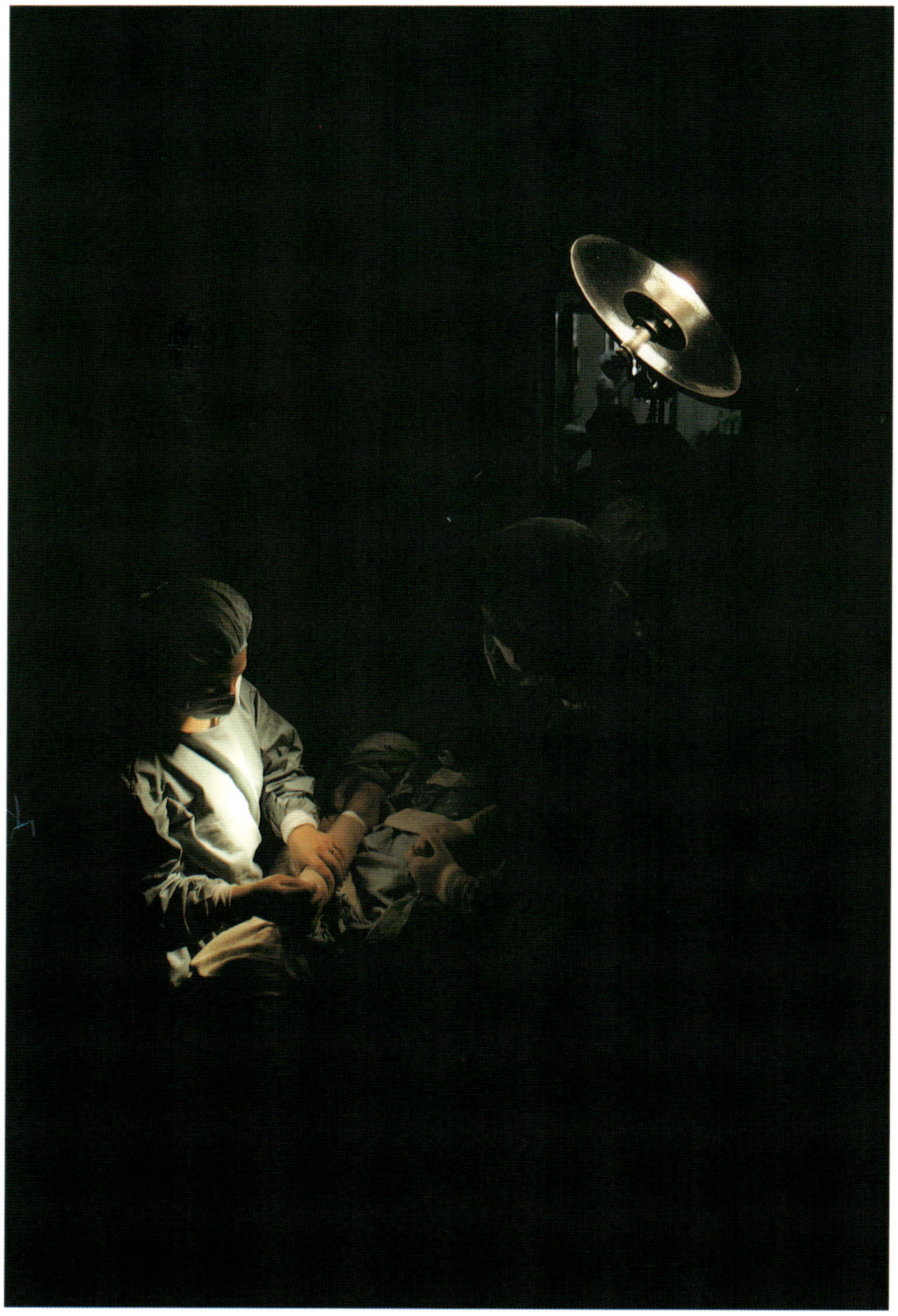

surgery, Hanoi

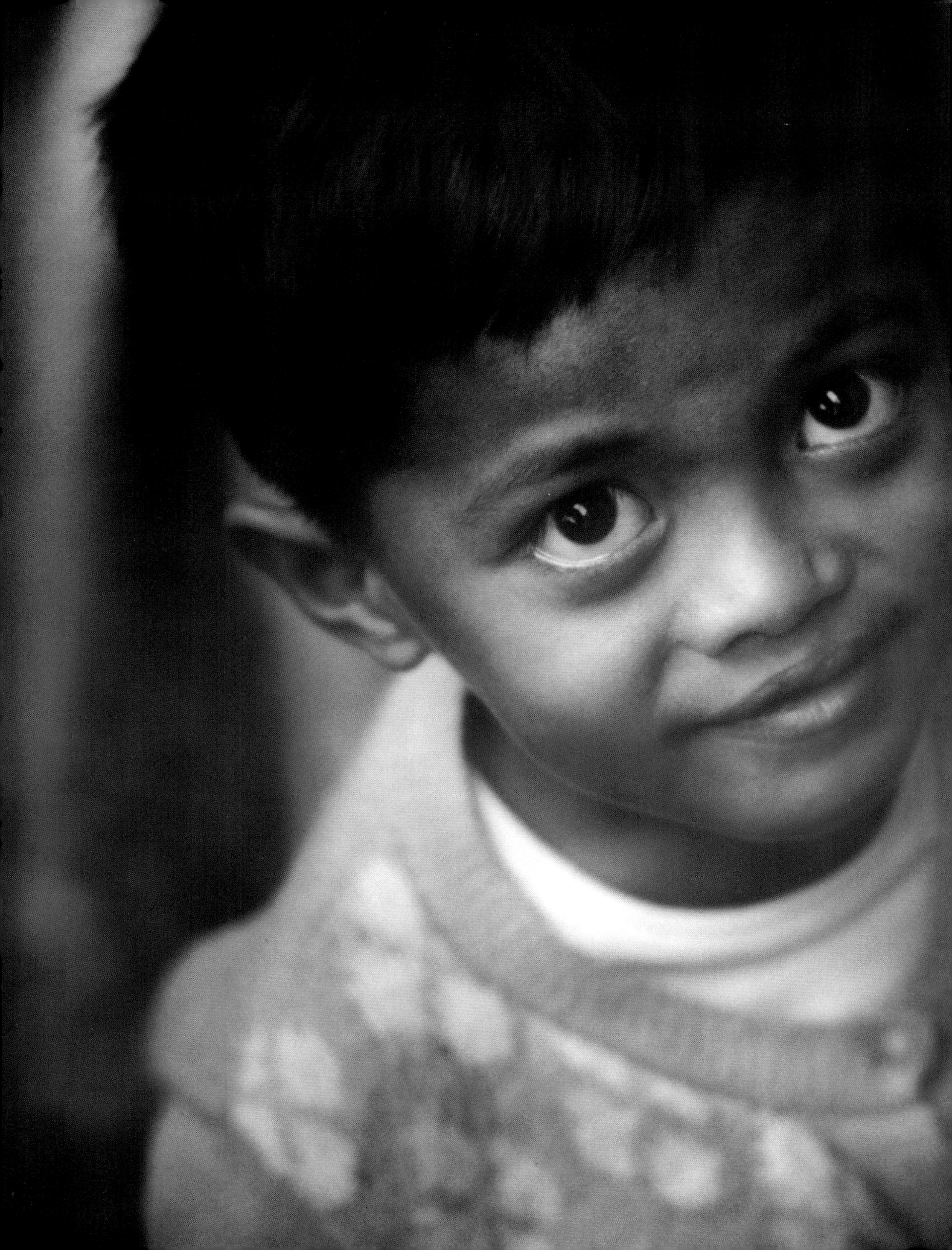

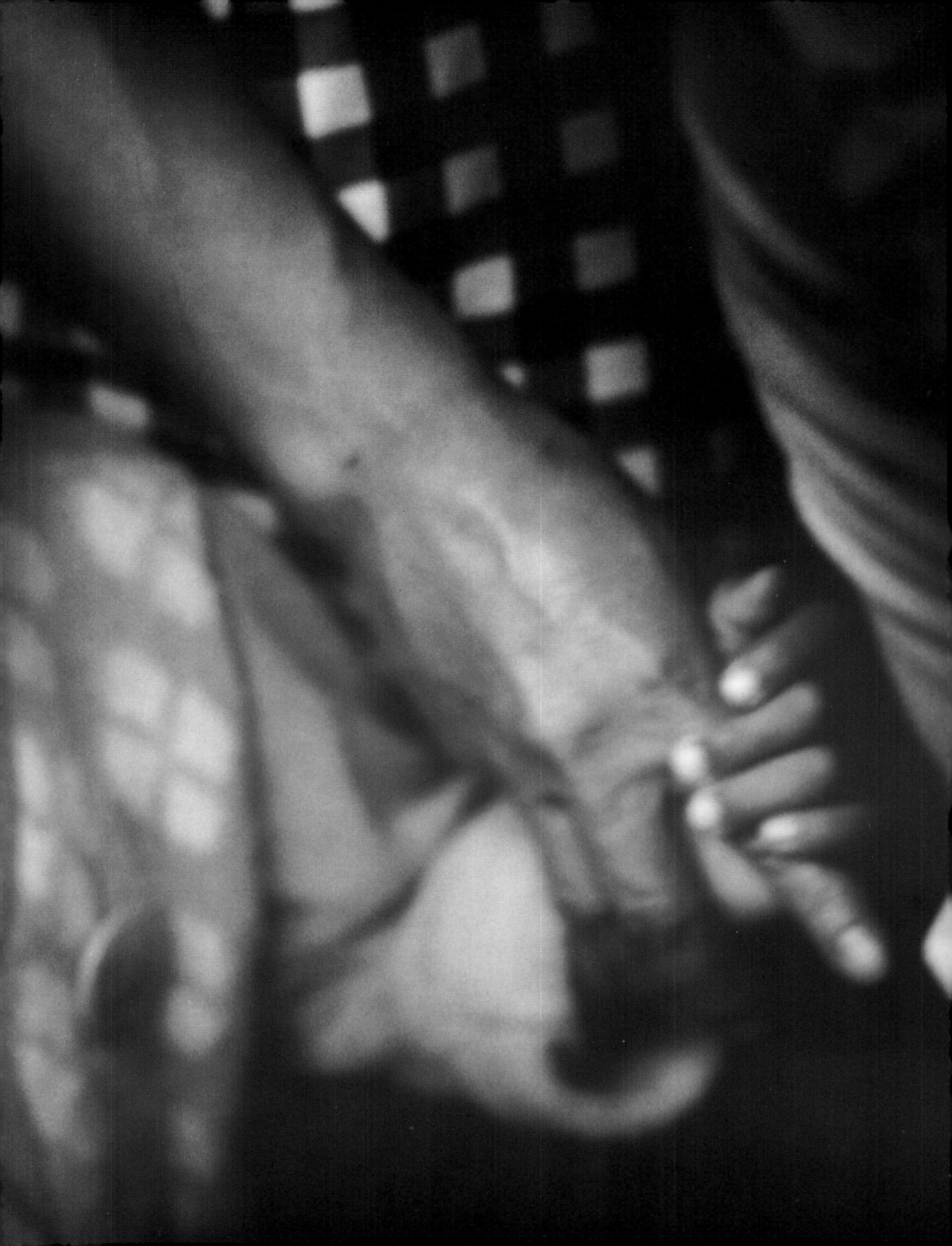

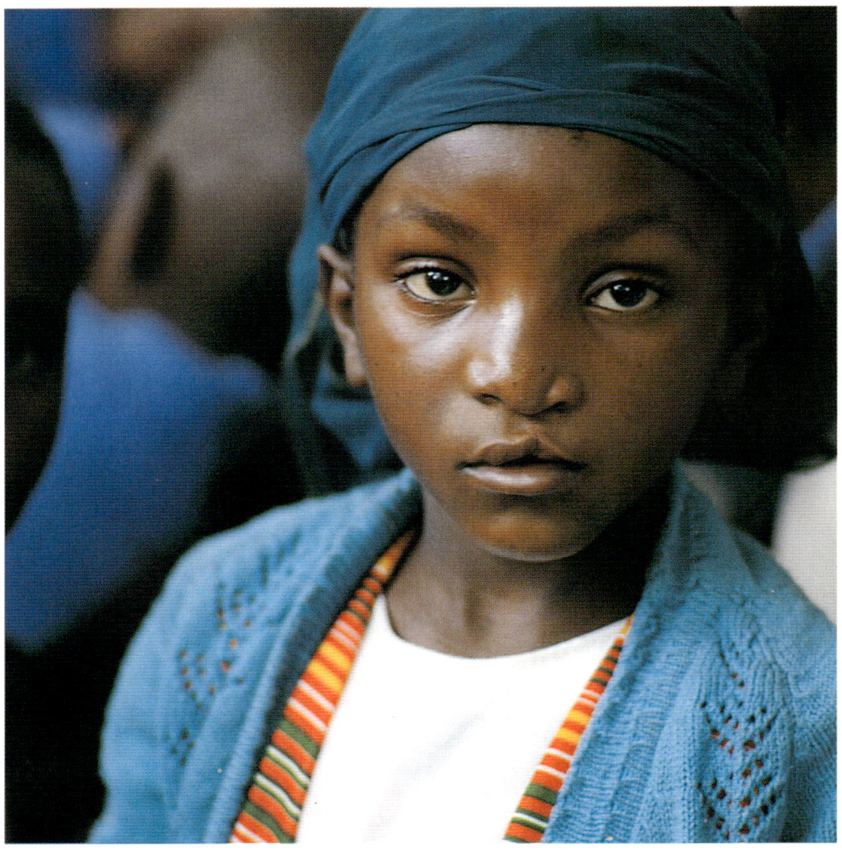

girl awaiting treatment, Nairobi
(previous spread) boy at screening, Naga City

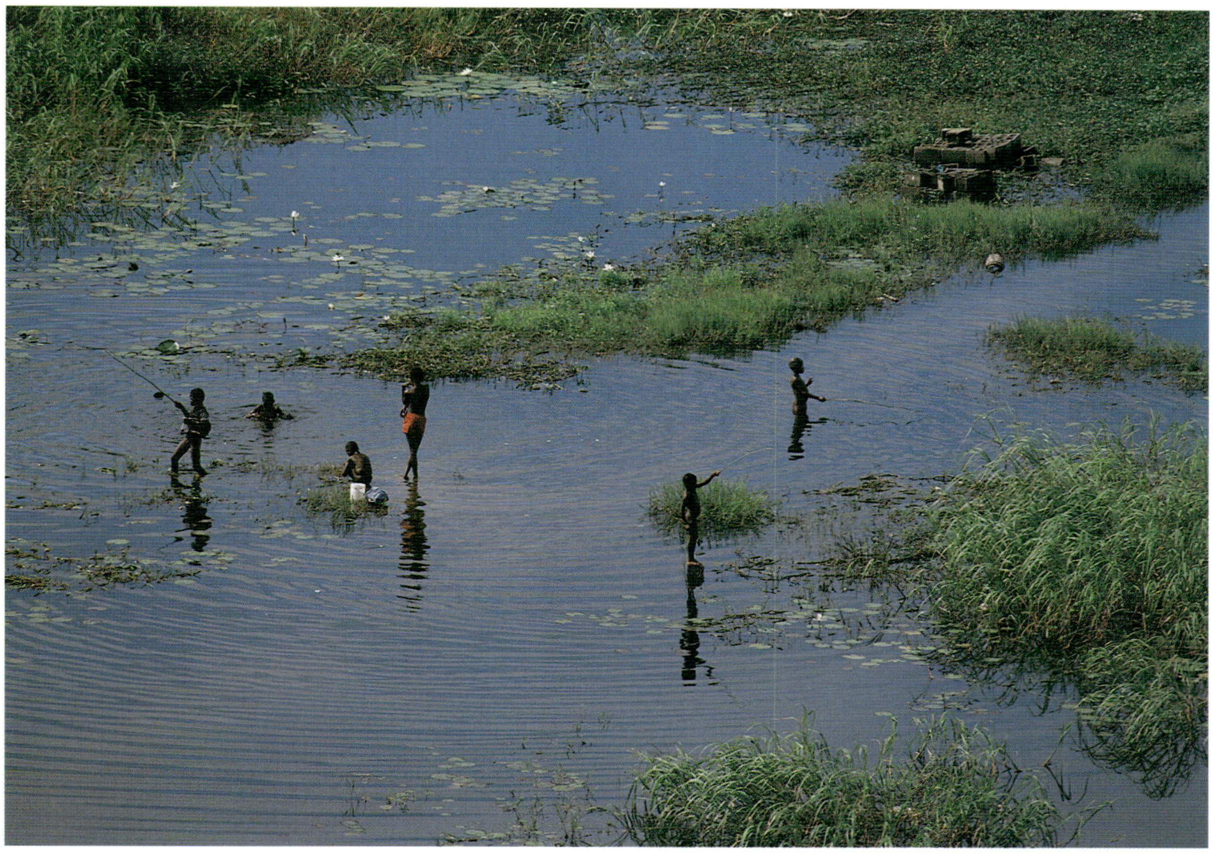

children playing behind hospital, Monrovia

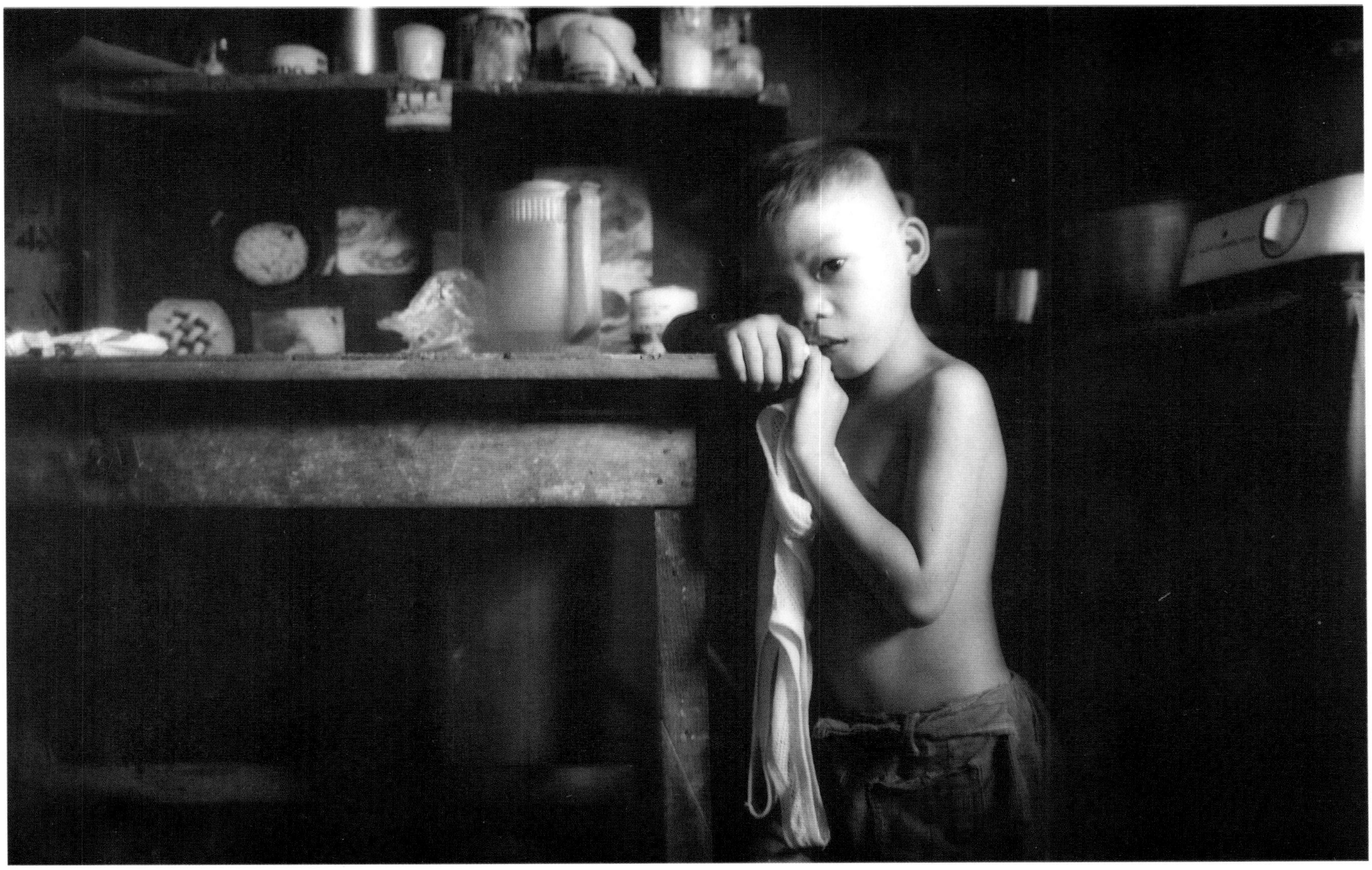

boy at Metro Manila dump

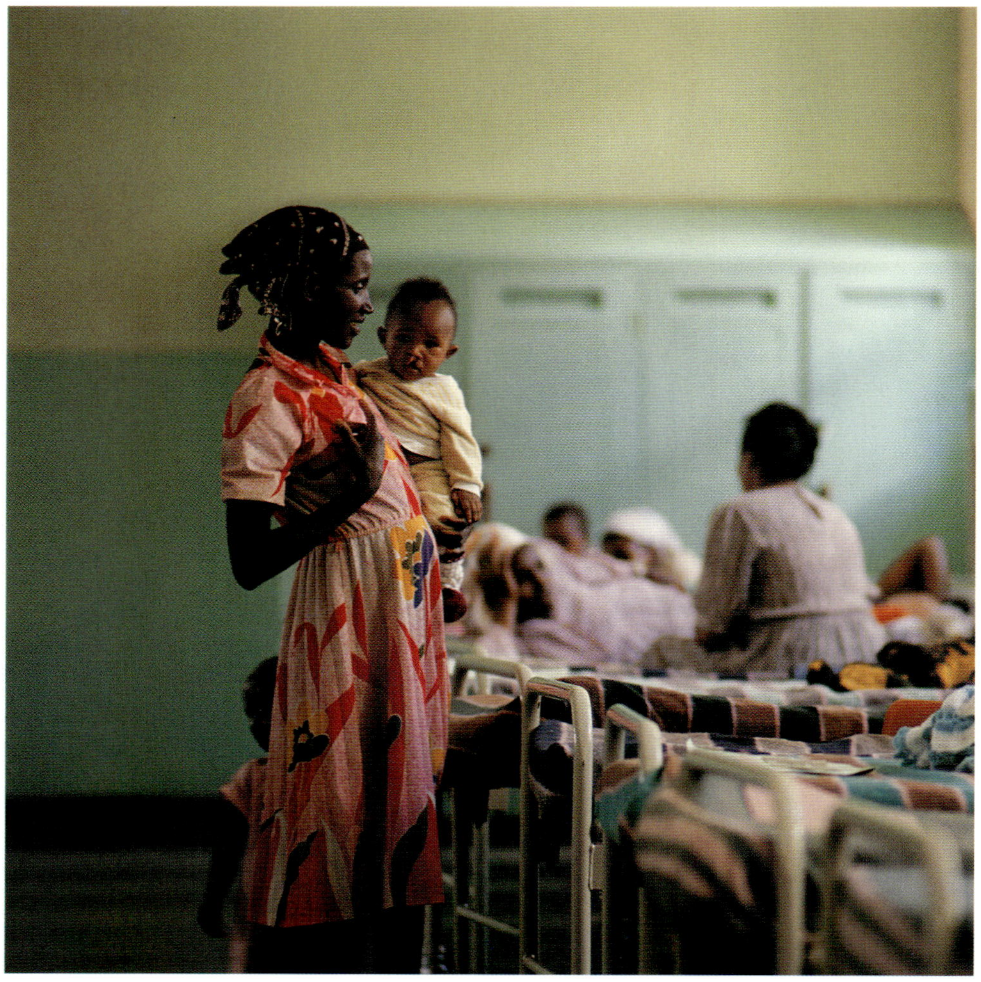

families and children on hospital ward, Nairobi
facing page photograph by Barbara Kinney

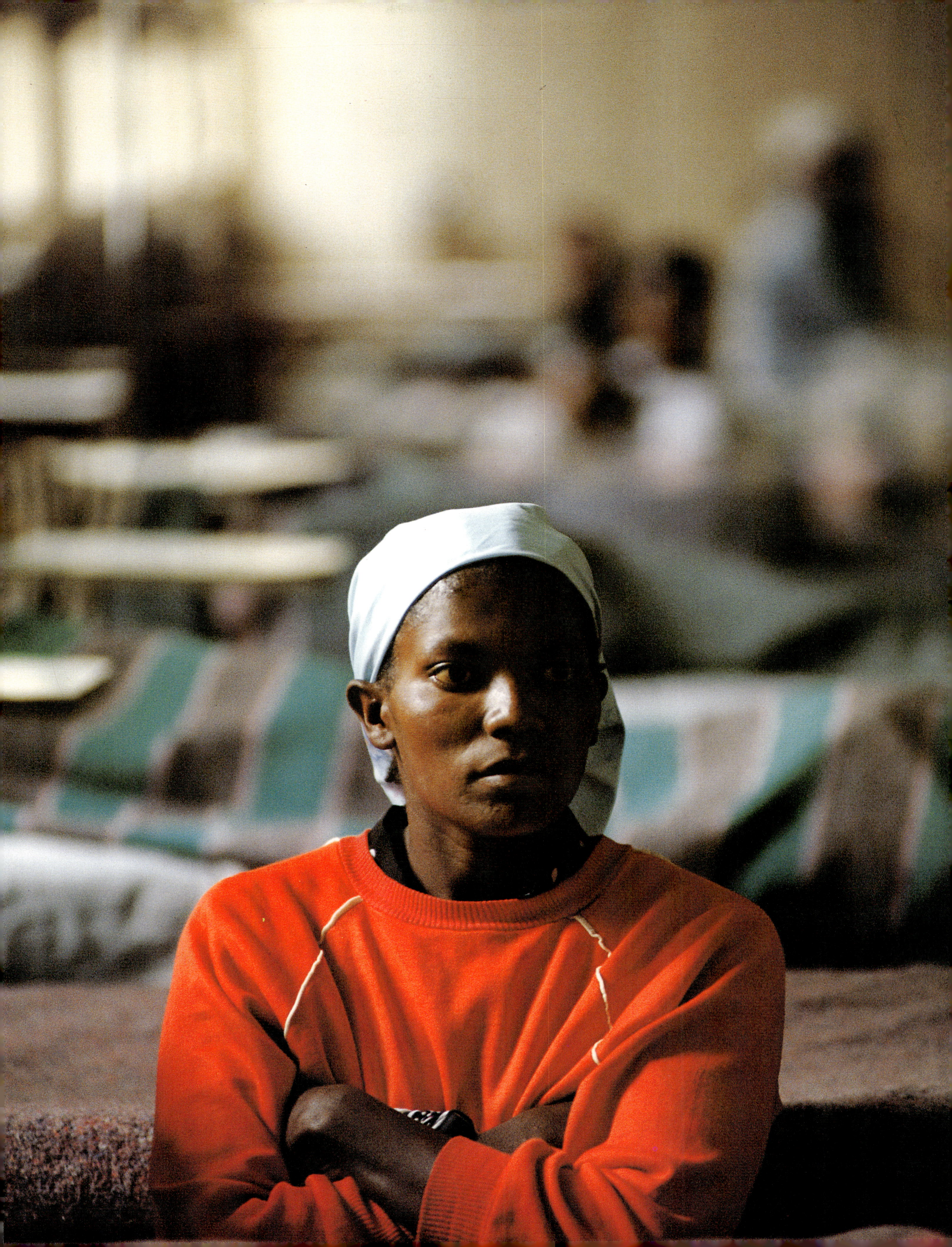

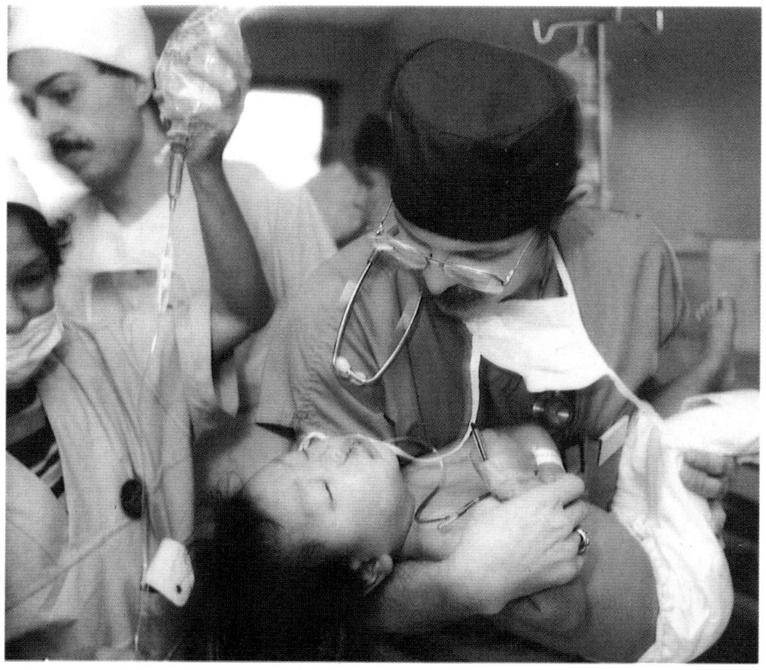

anesthesiologist with child in pre-op, Hanoi

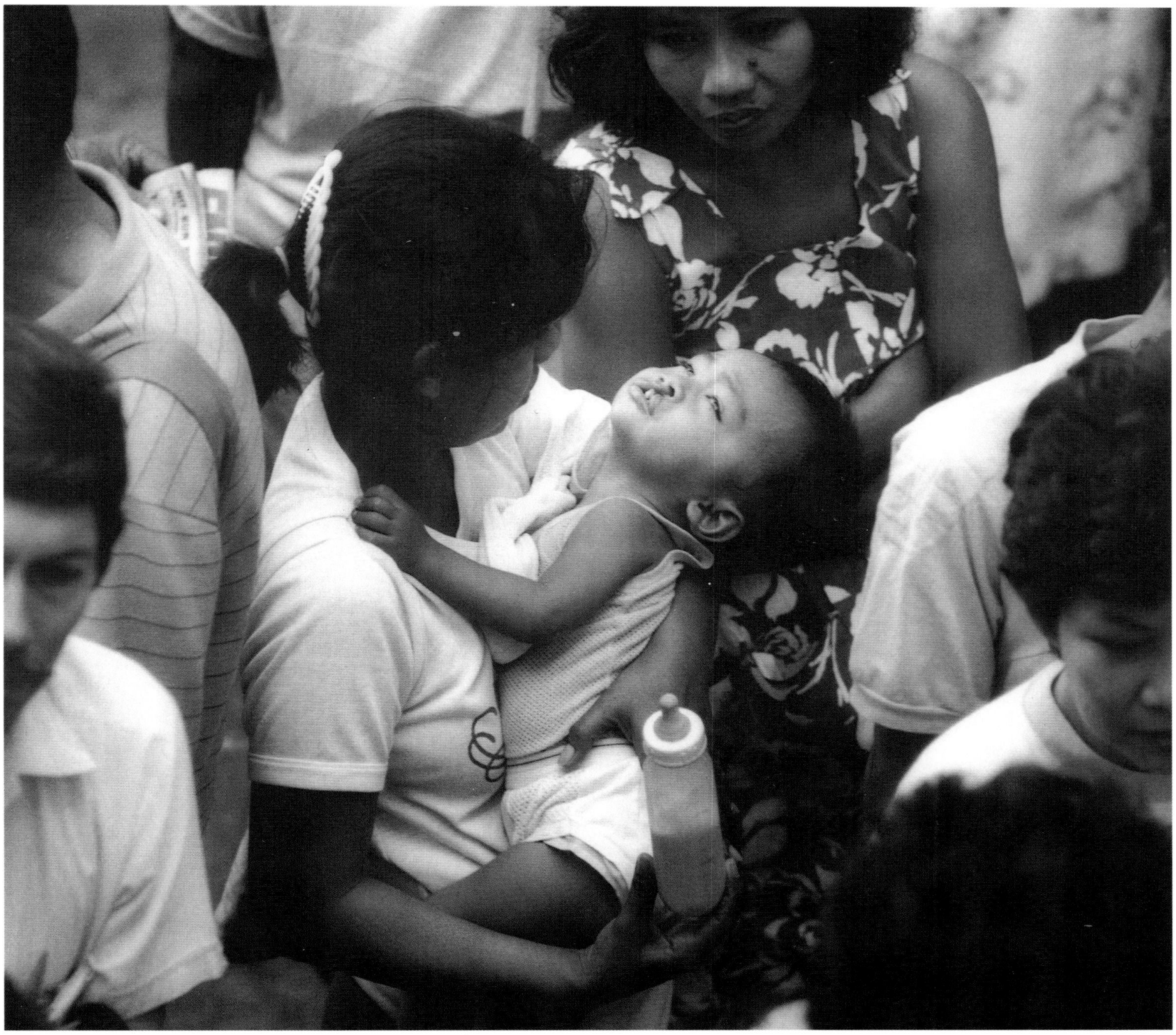

families and children outside hospital, Manila

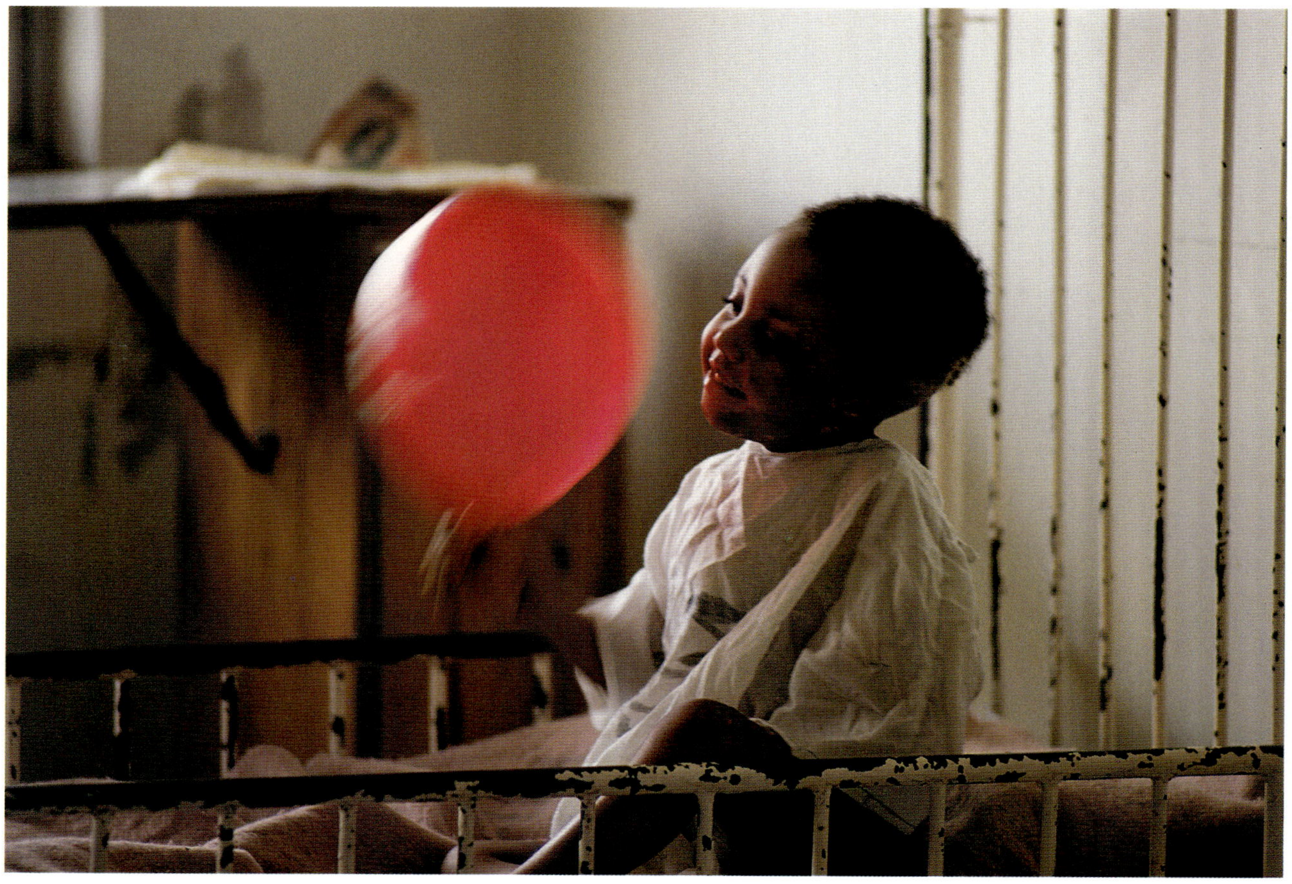

boy and balloon, Nairobi

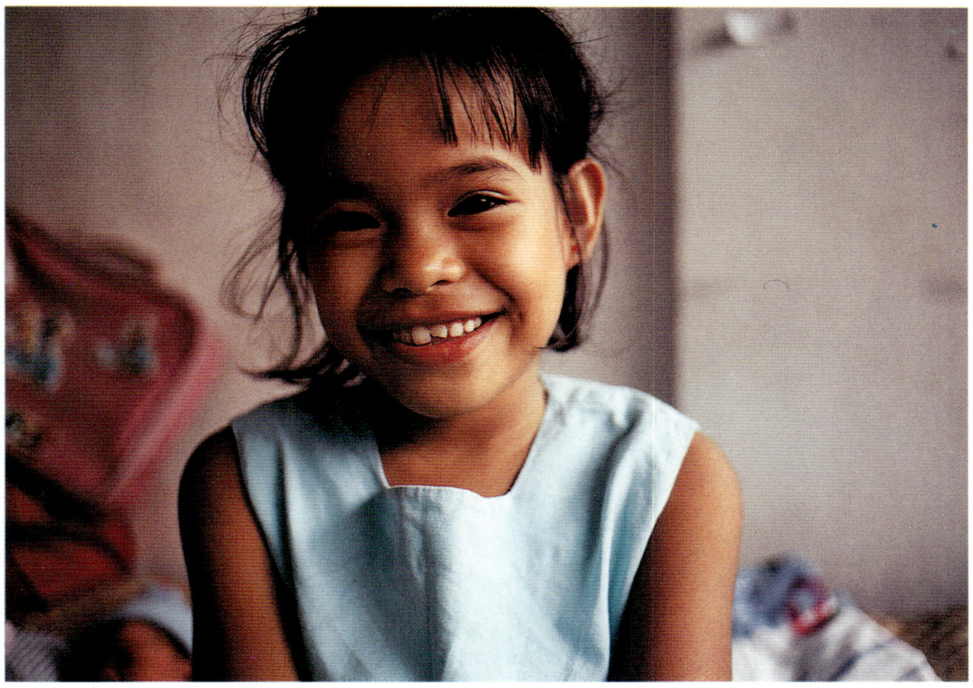

girl on children's ward, Panama City

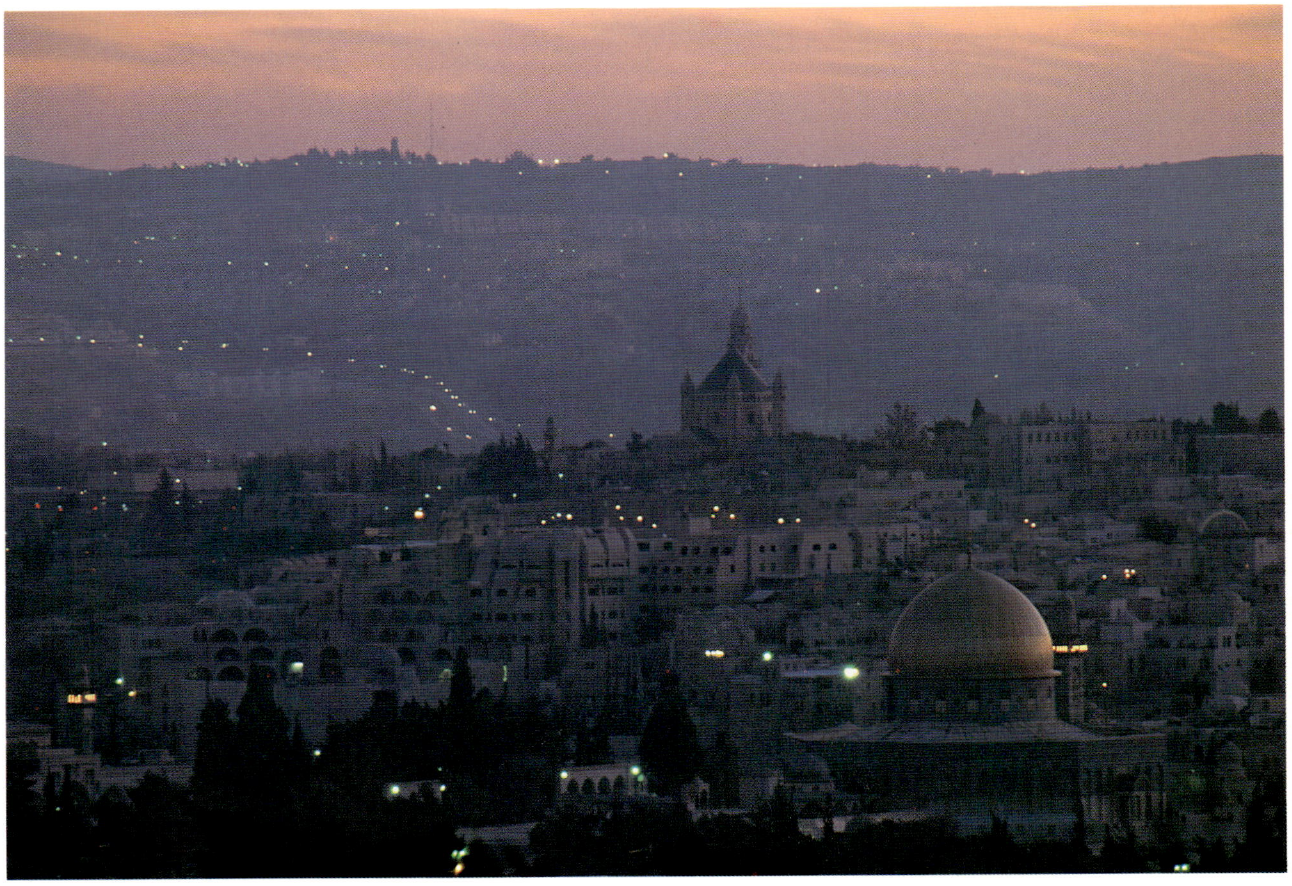

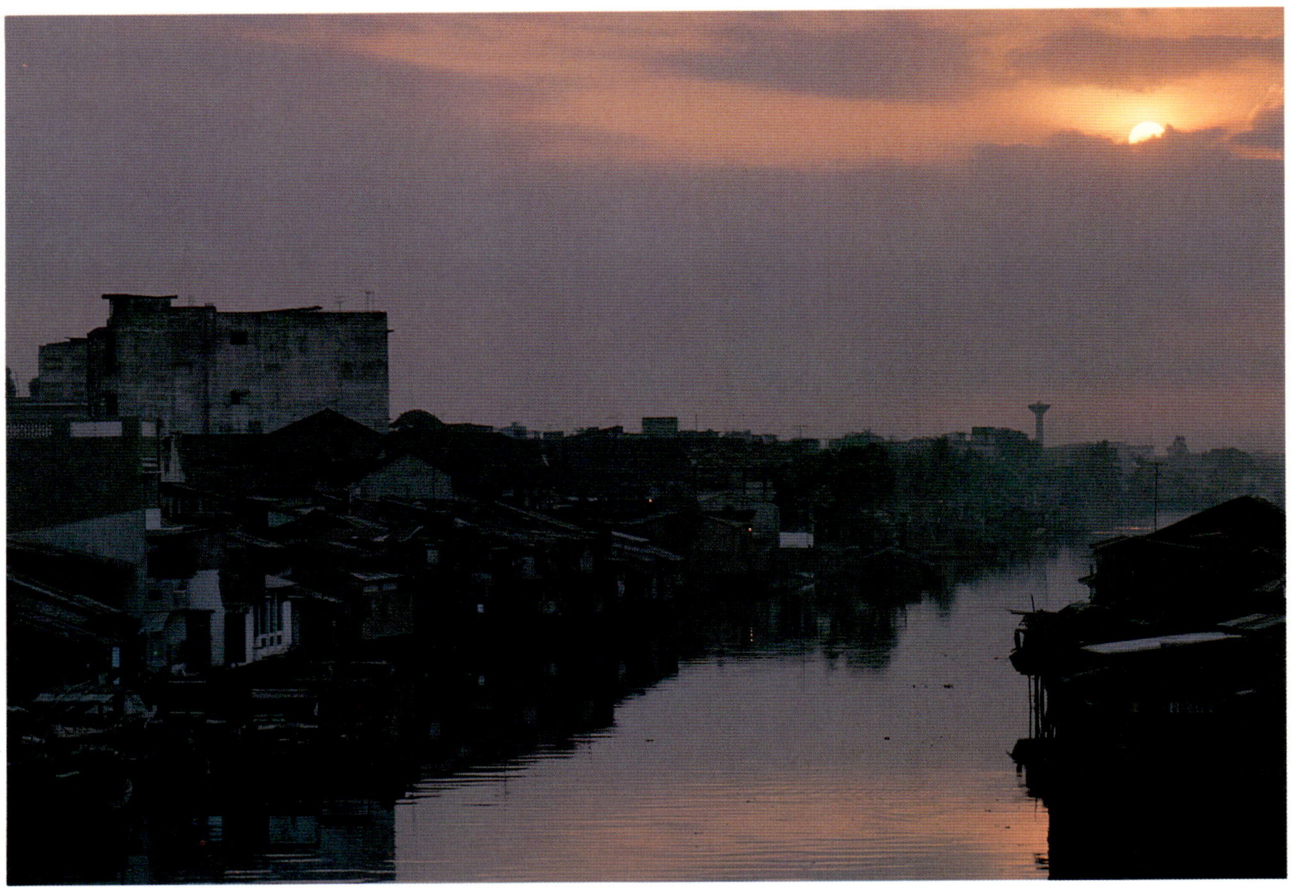

sunsets, Jerusalem and Saigon

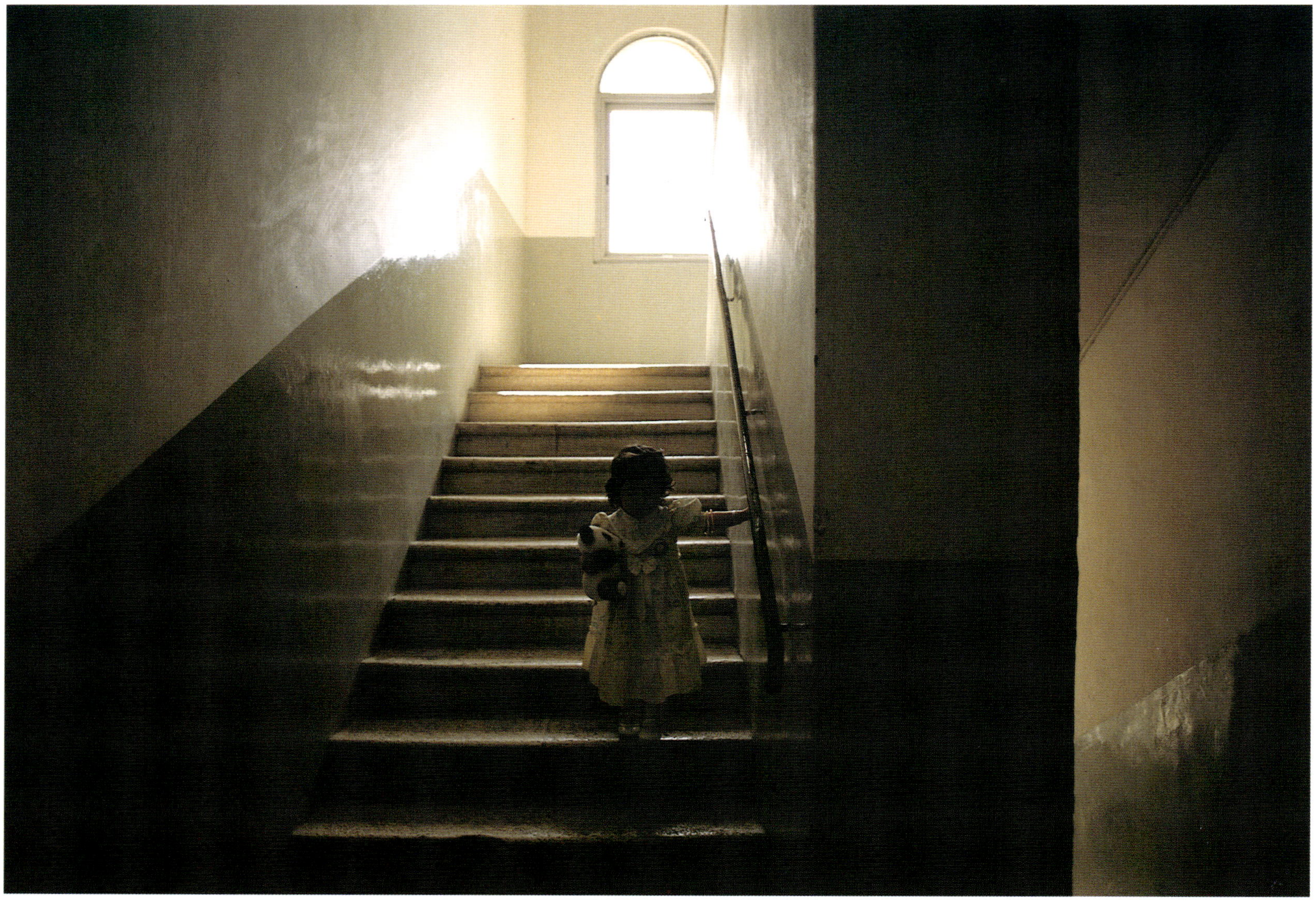

girl in stairwell, Jerusalem

Much to the delight of parents and volunteers,
cherubic cheeks and rosebud lips
would occasionally part in a coaxed smile.

MORTON H. GOLDSTEIN, MD
OSI MEDICAL VOLUNTEER

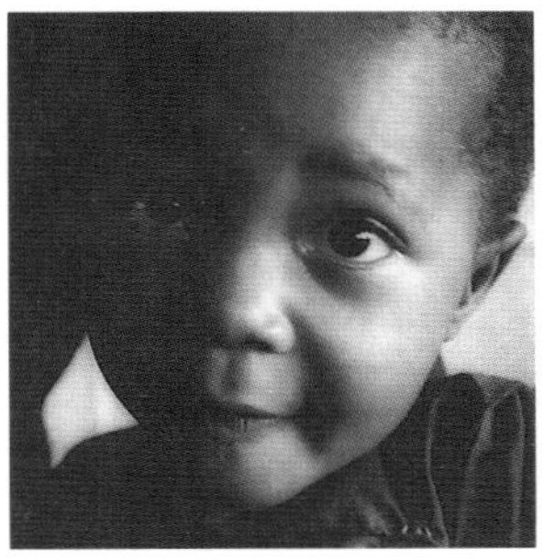

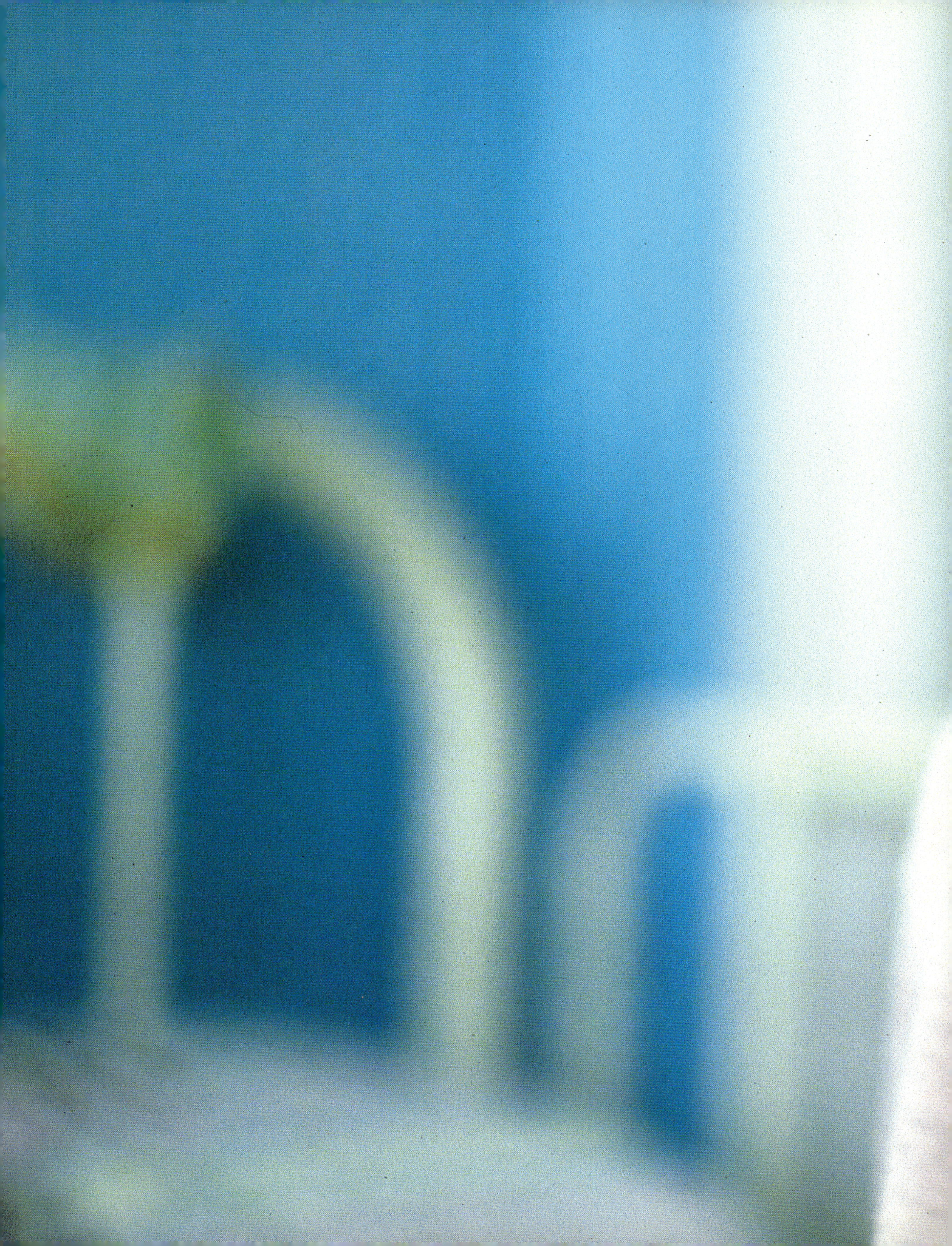

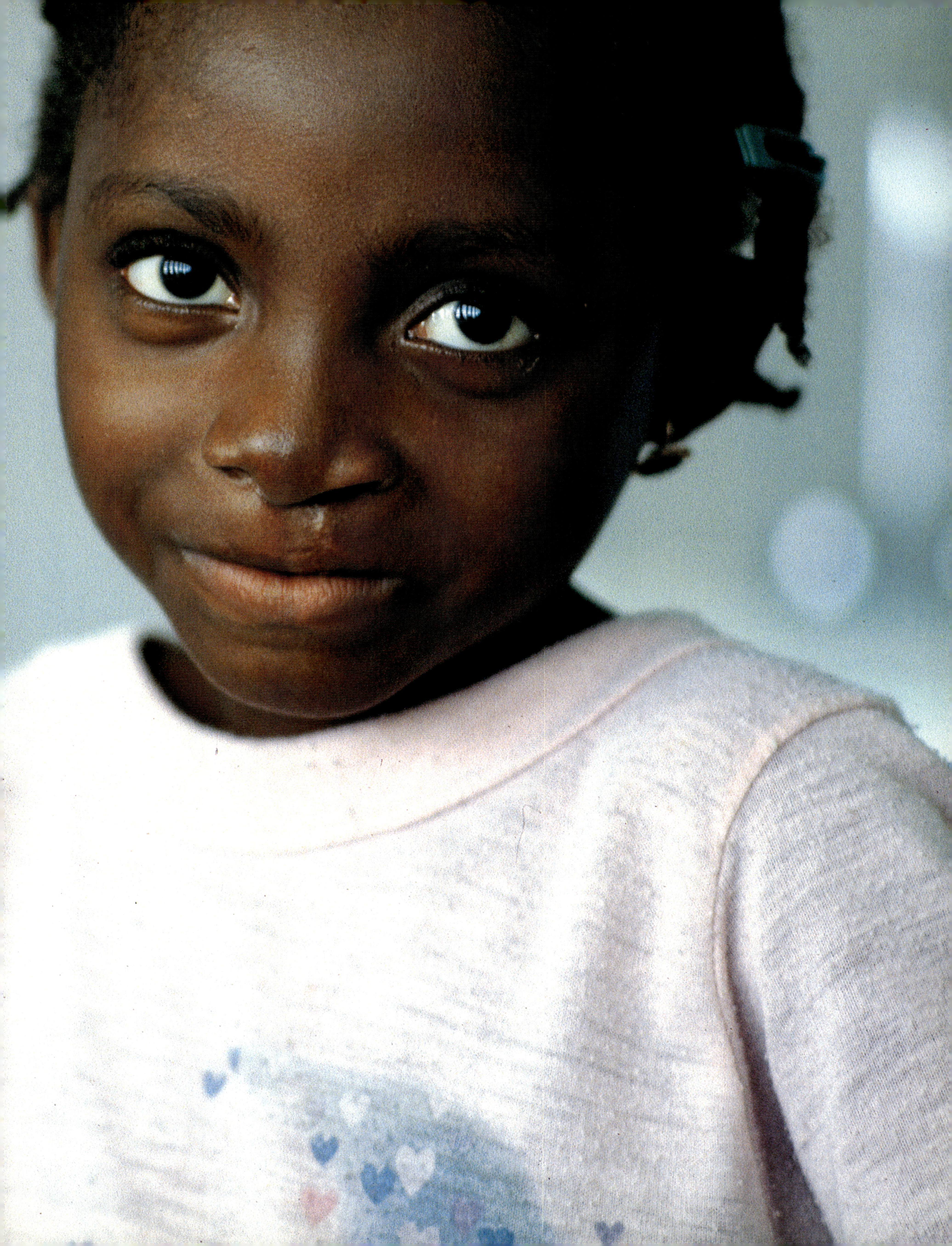

(previous spread) girl in hospital, Monrovia

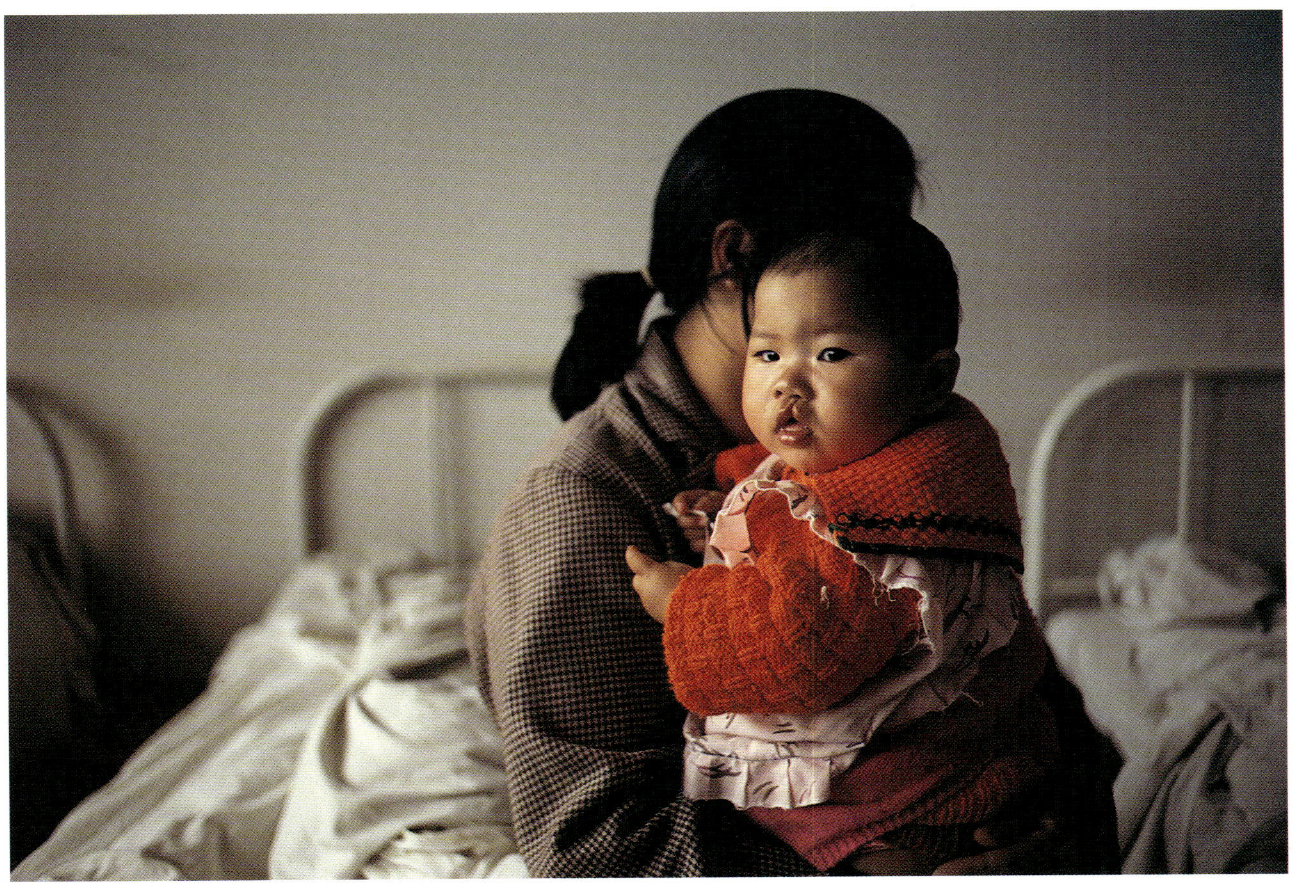

mother and child in pre-op, Hangzhou

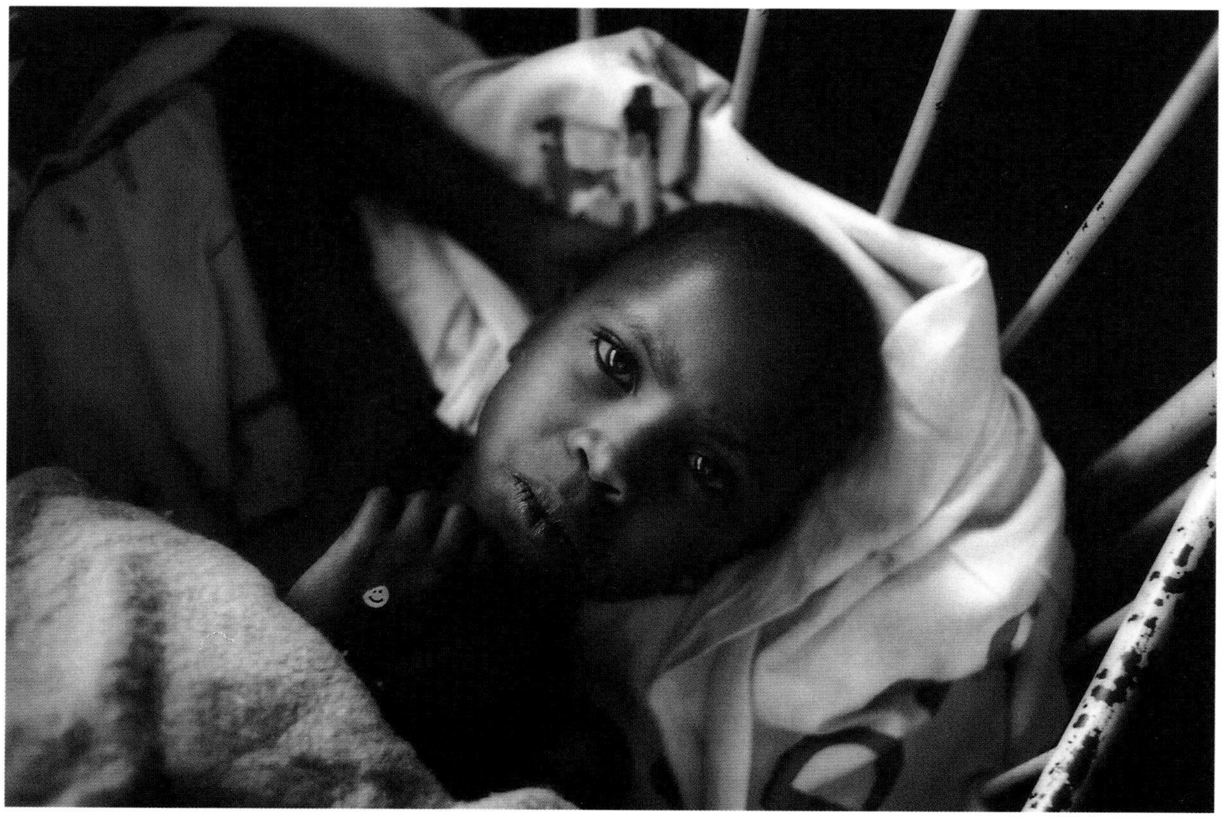

boy in hospital bed, Nairobi

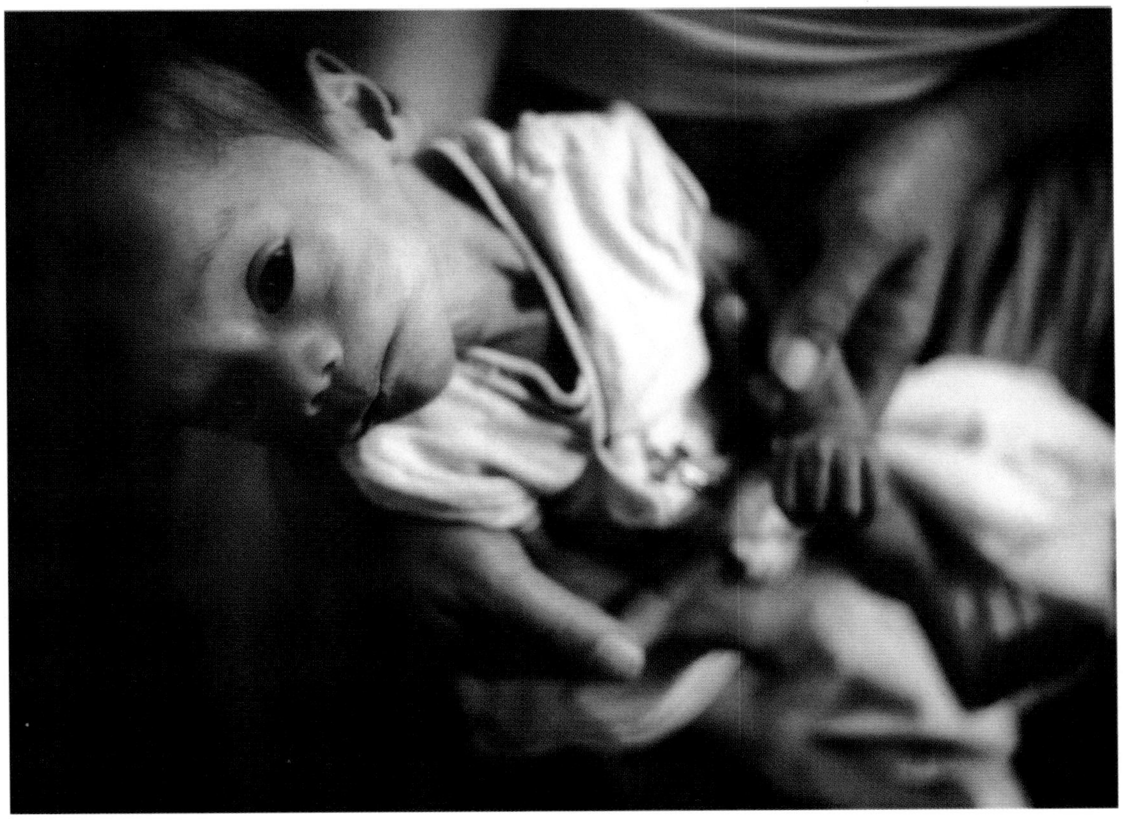

malnourished child, Negros

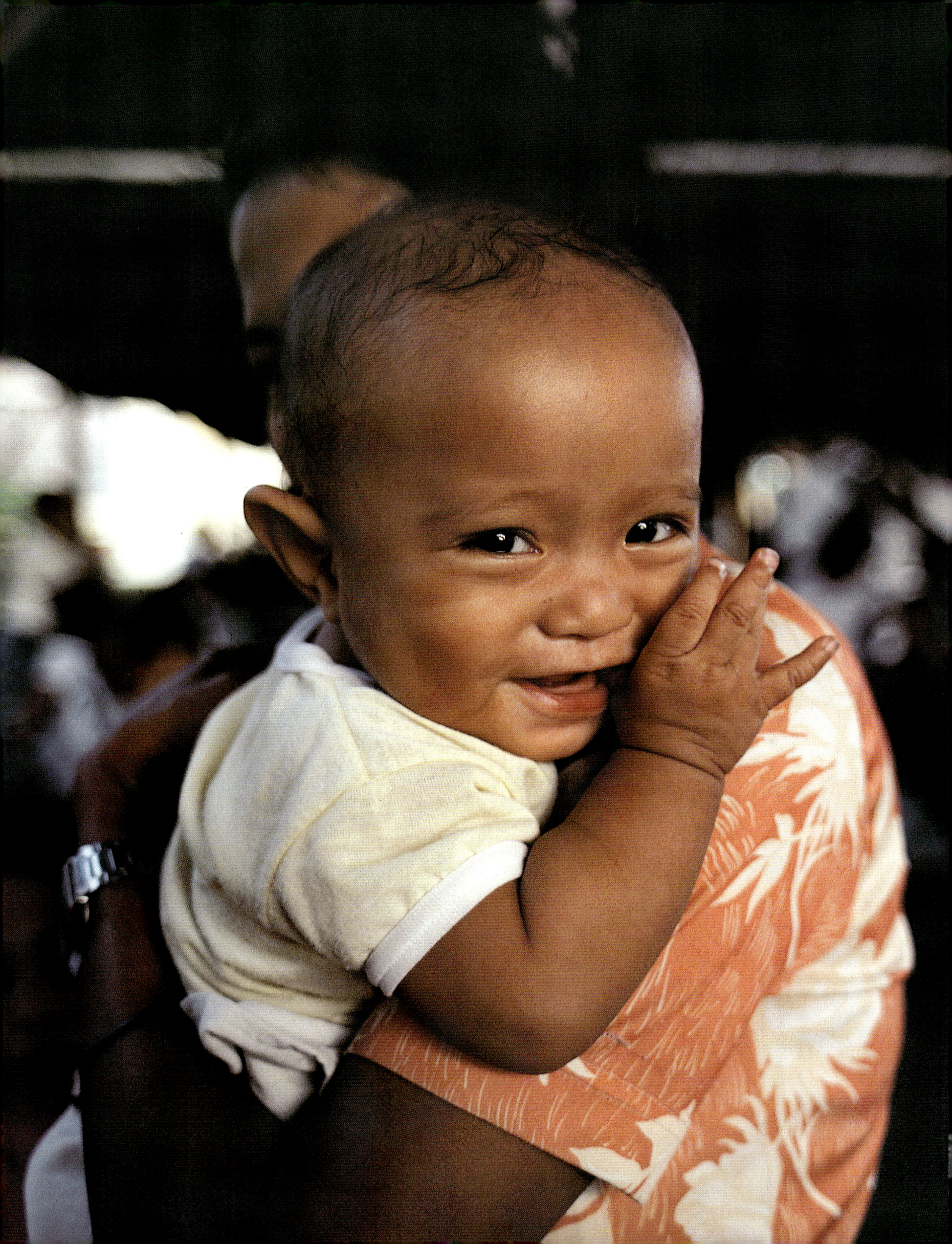

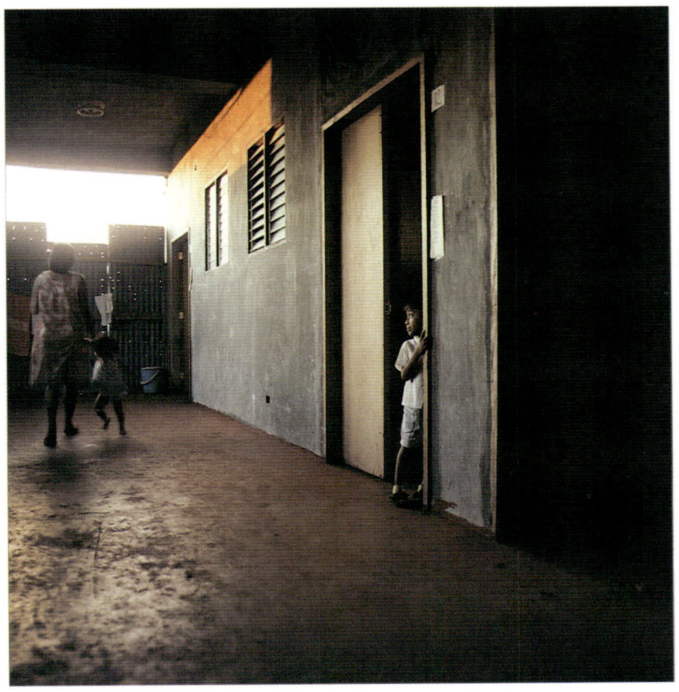

boy and mother await screening, Naga City
skipping in the hospital hallway, Naga City

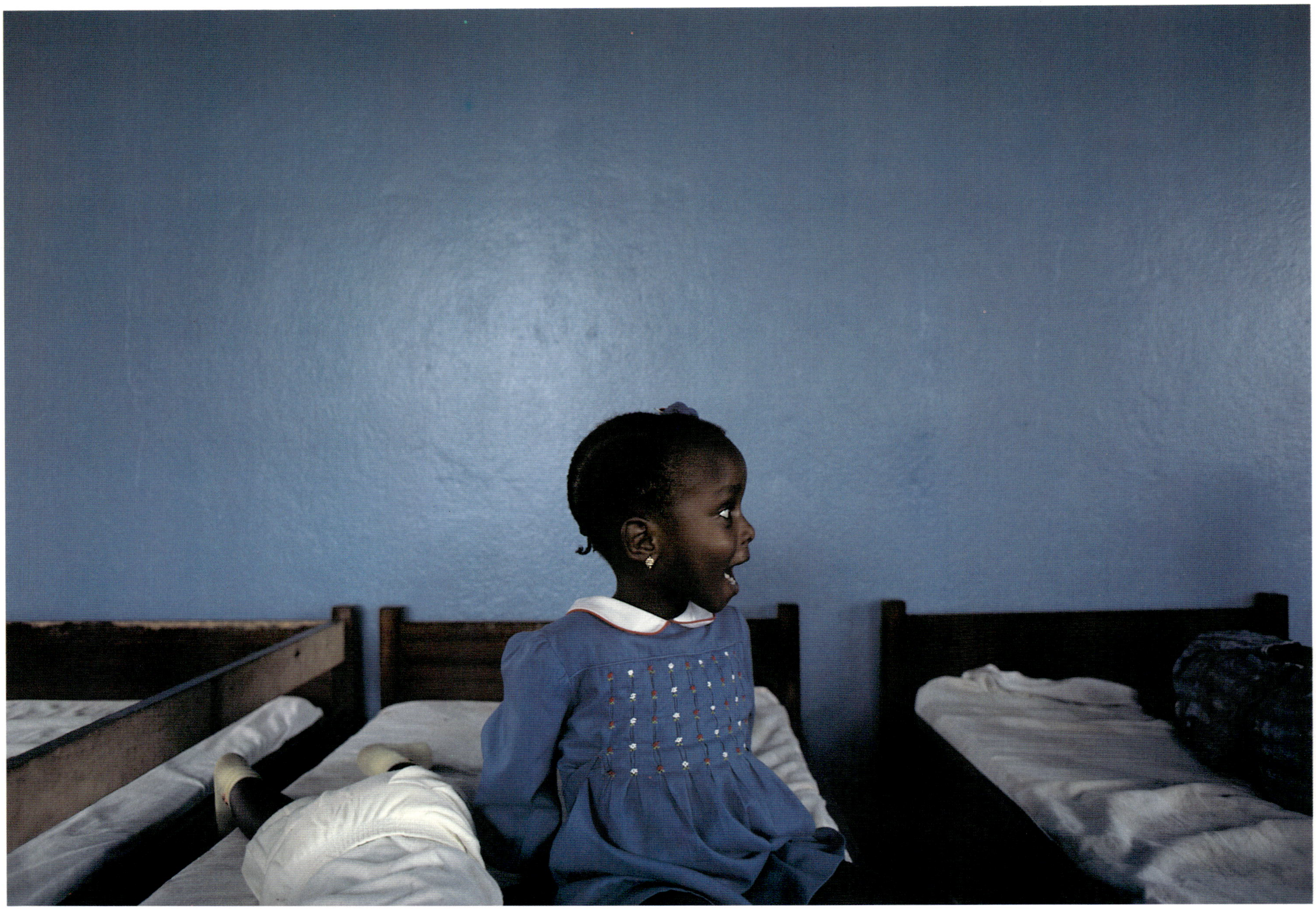

girl in blue dress, Monrovia

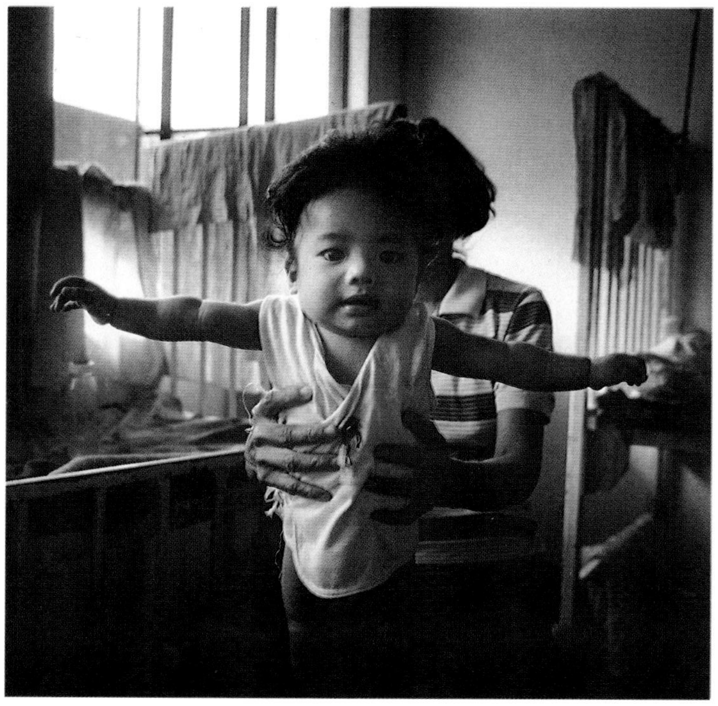

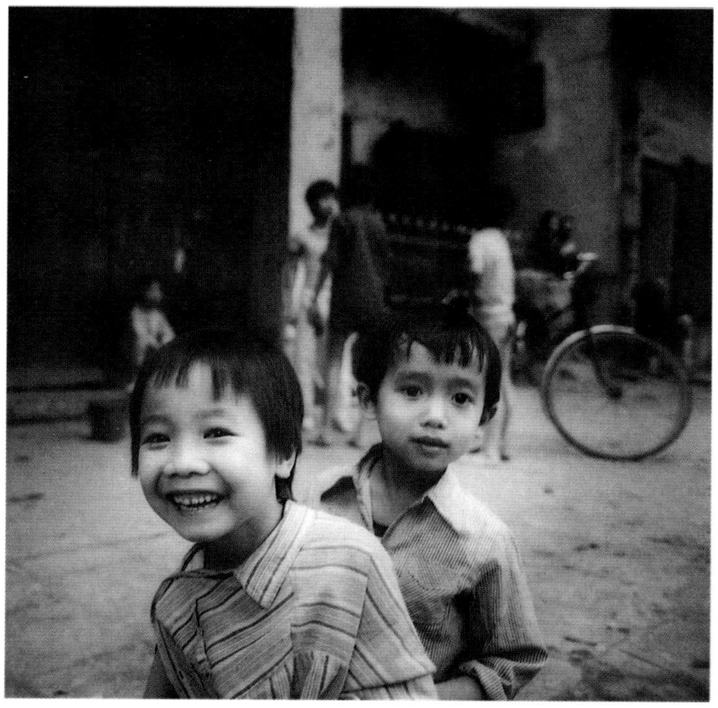

children, Negros and Saigon

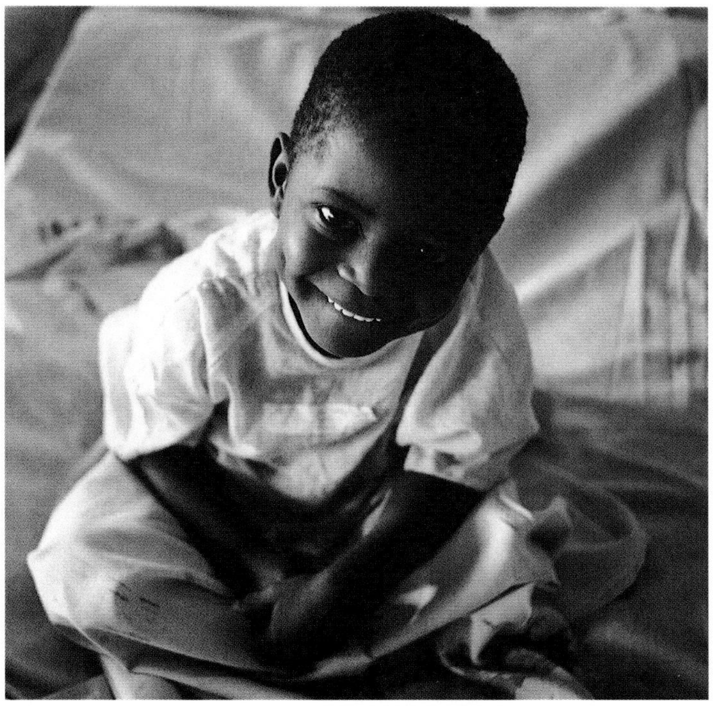

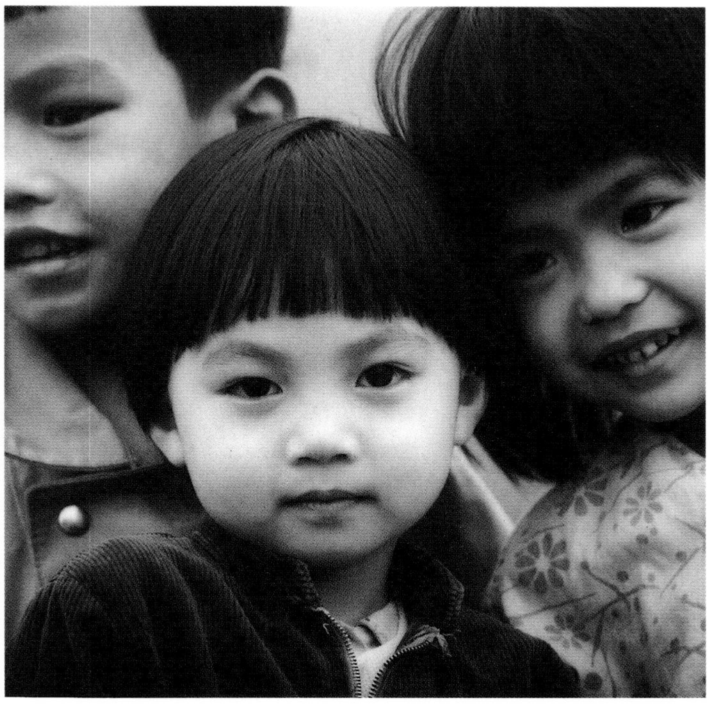

children, Nairobi and Hanoi

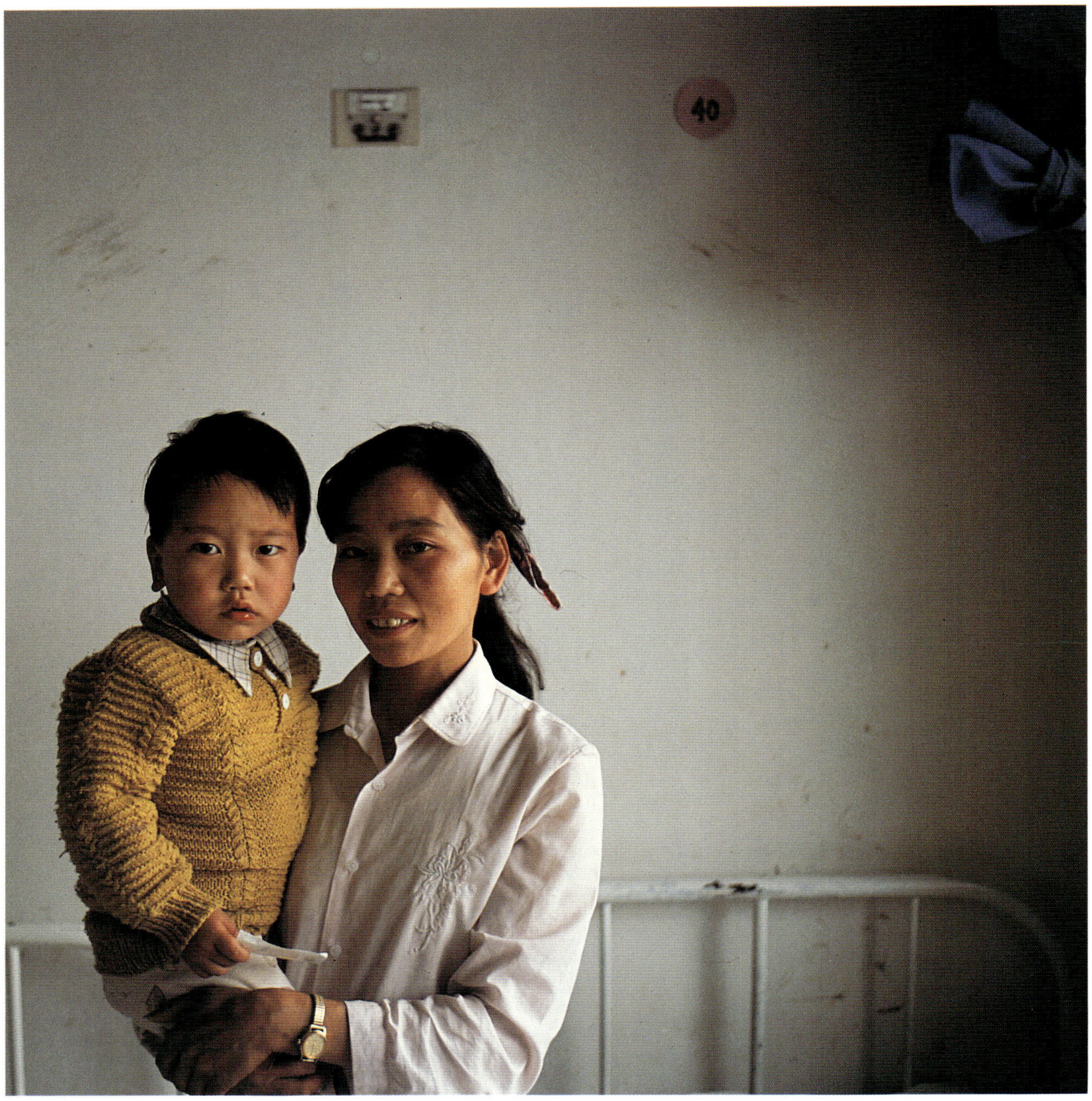

mother and child, Hangzhou

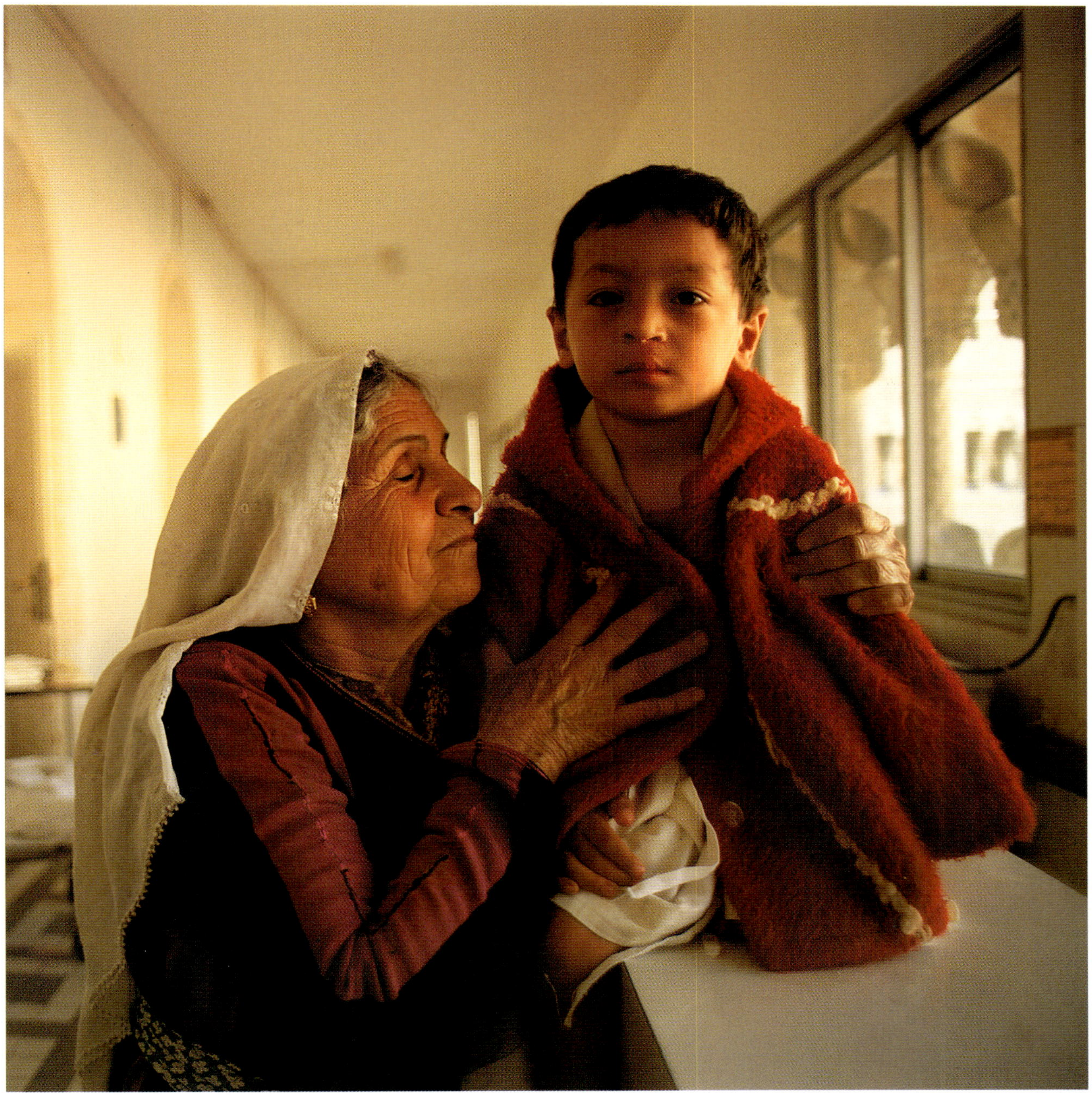

boy and grandmother, Jerusalem

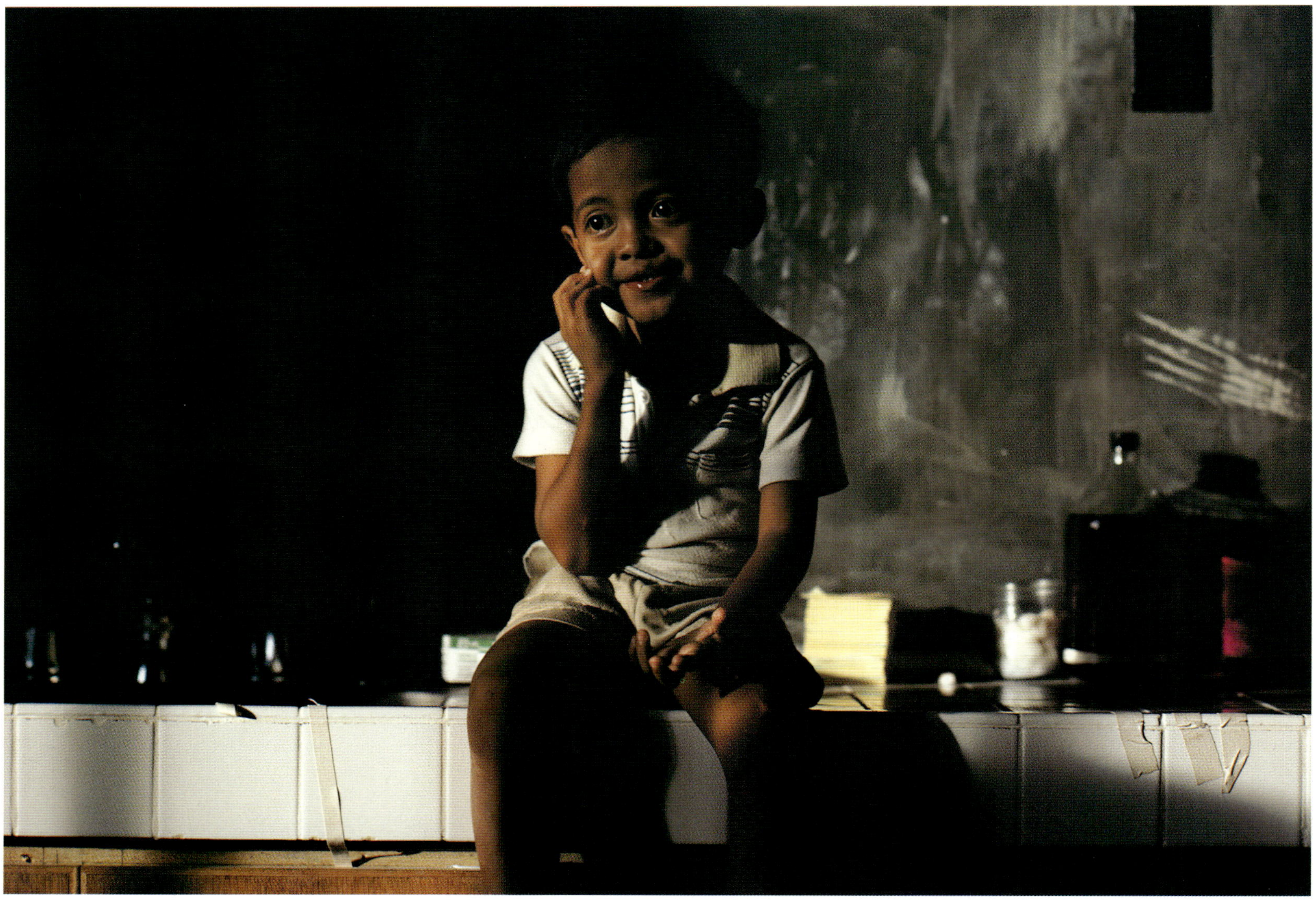

boy on the counter, Naga City

Operation Smile is a small bridge to peace.
It's certainly not always an easy one to build or cross.
Forged from the sweat, tears, love and sacrifice, and very hard work of countless people, it is a bridge built for, and dedicated to, the children of the world.

It cannot be allowed to fail, ever.

NORMAN THOMAS SCOTT, MD
OSI MEDICAL VOLUNTEER

(following spread) girl in hospital hallway, Jerusalem

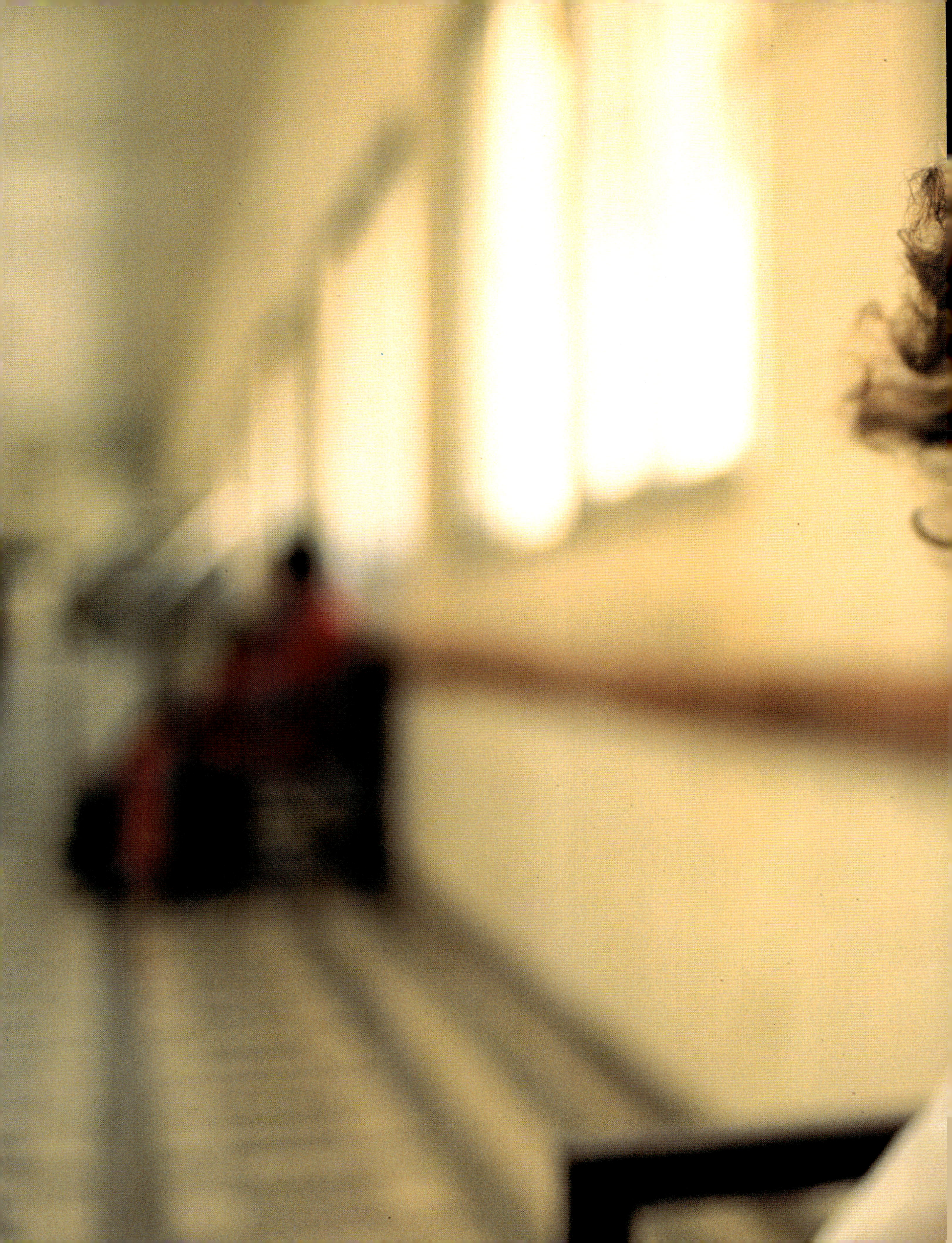

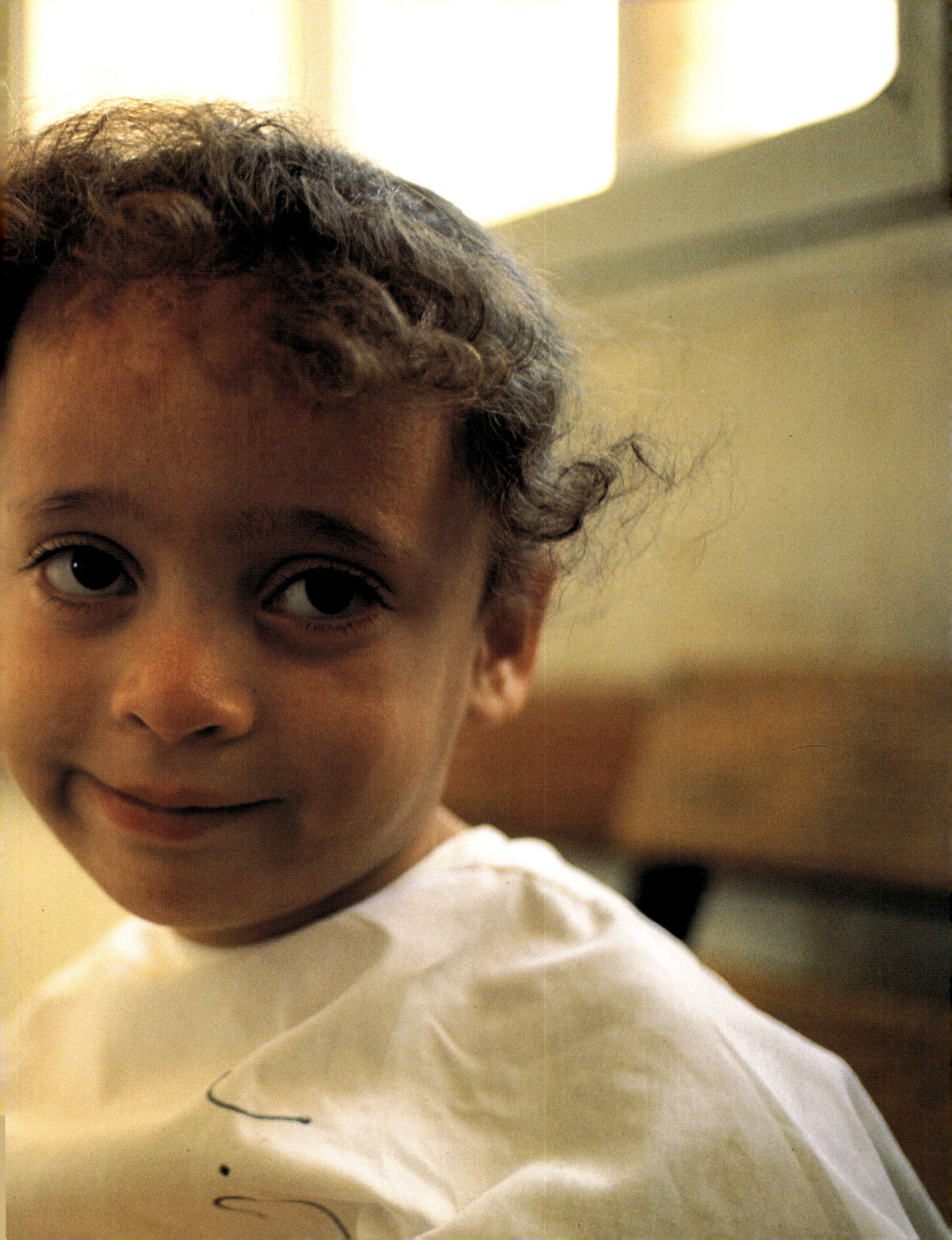

CHRONOLOGY

1982

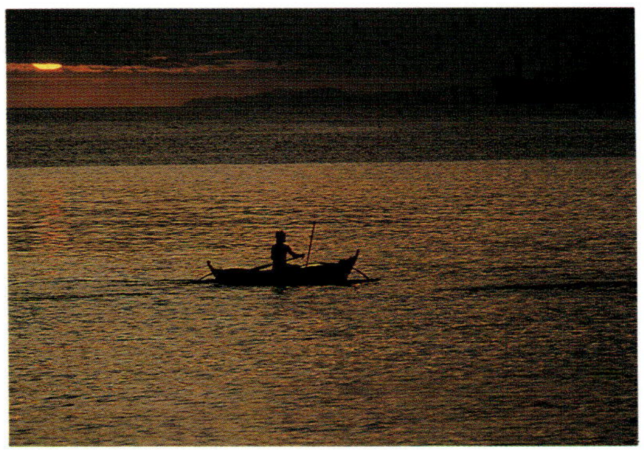

November	Naga City, Philippines

1984

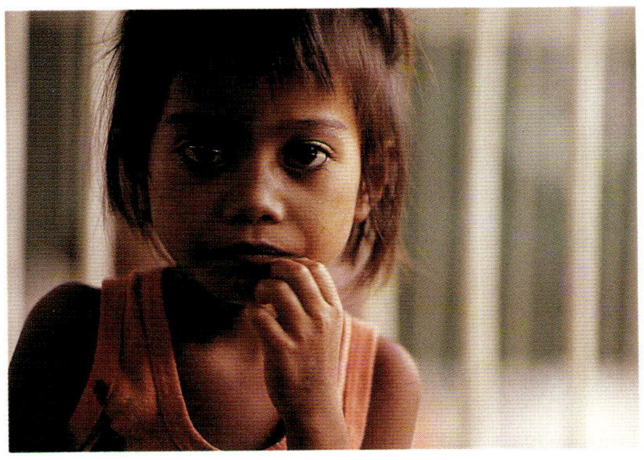

February	Naga City, Philippines

1985

February	Naga City, Philippines

1986

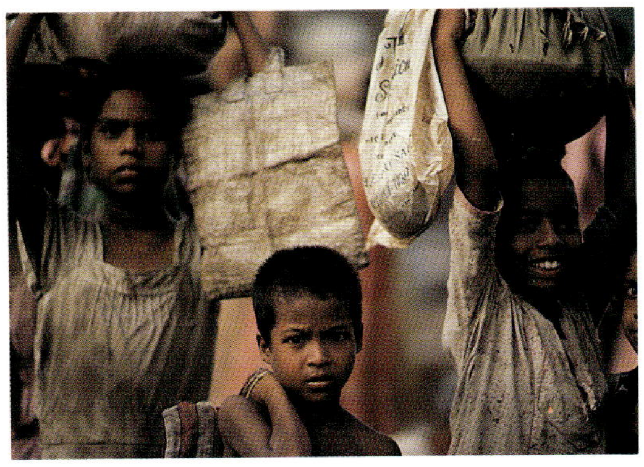

February	Naga City, Philippines Manila, Philippines Negros, Philippines
May	Nairobi, Kenya Monrovia, Liberia Calcutta, India

1987

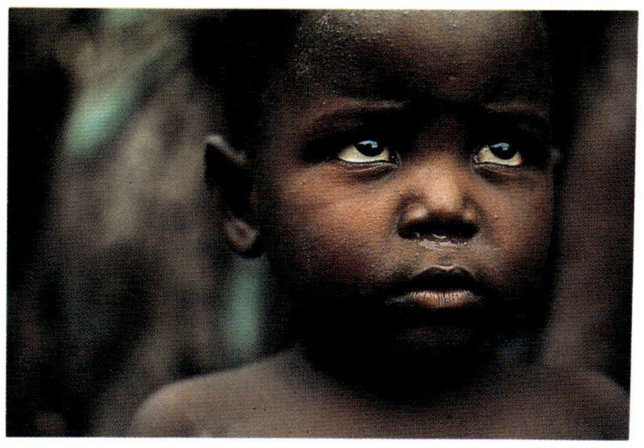

February	Naga City, Philippines Manila, Philippines Negros, Philippines
June	Manizales, Colombia
September	Monrovia, Liberia Nairobi, Kenya

1988

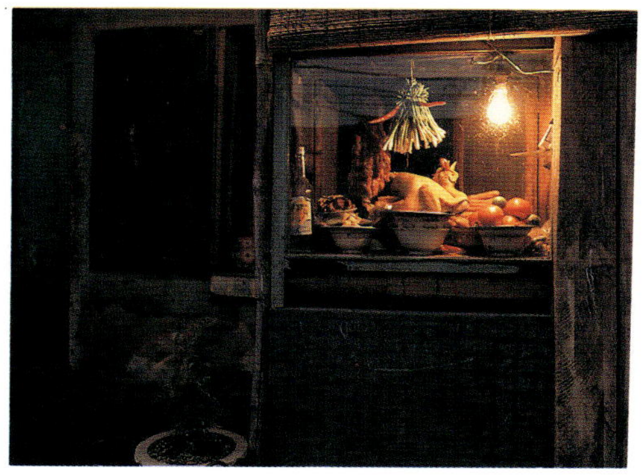

February	Naga City, Philippines Manila, Philippines Negros, Philippines
June	Manizales, Colombia
August	Hanoi, Vietnam Saigon, Vietnam
September	Monrovia, Liberia Nairobi, Kenya

1989

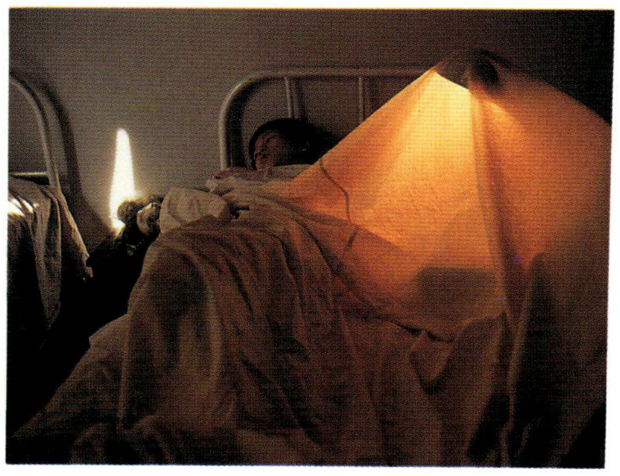

February	Naga City, Philippines Manila, Philippines Negros, Philippines Hanoi, Vietnam
July	Manizales, Colombia
October	Monrovia, Liberia Nairobi, Kenya Accra, Ghana

1990

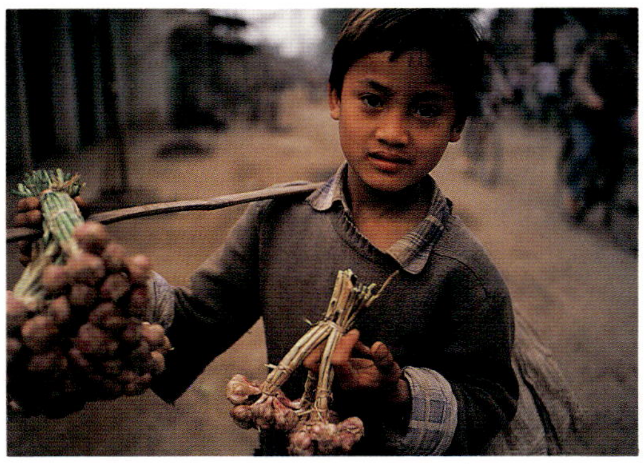

February	Naga City, Philippines Manila, Philippines Negros, Philippines
February	Hanoi, Vietnam Saigon, Vietnam
July	Nairobi, Kenya
September	Accra, Ghana
November	Manizales, Colombia

1991

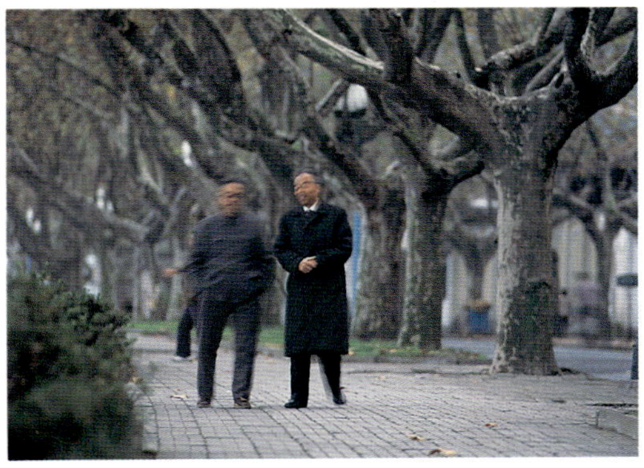

January	Panama City, Panama
February	Naga City, Philippines Manila, Philippines Negros, Philippines
May	Hangzhou, China
July	Panama City, Panama
September	Nairobi, Kenya Bucharest, Romania
November	Hanoi, Vietnam Hue City, Vietnam Manizales, Colombia

1992

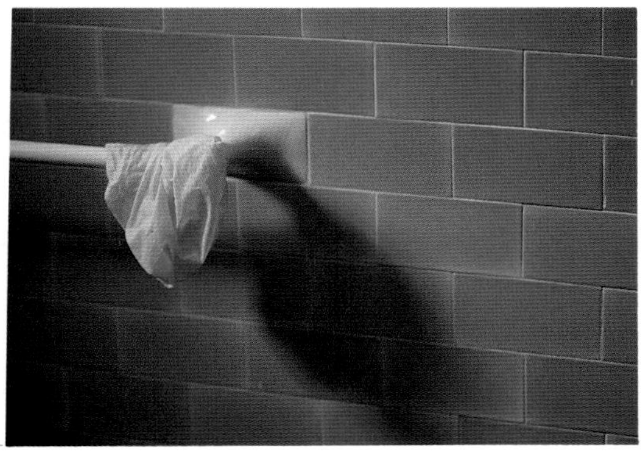

February	Naga City, Philippines Manila, Philippines Negros, Philippines
March	East Jerusalem, Israel Managua, Nicaragua
April	Hangzhou, China
July	Panama City, Panama David, Panama Caracas, Venezuela
September	St. Petersburg, Russia Nairobi, Kenya Kisumu, Kenya Bucharest, Romania
October	Meizhou, China Manizales, Colombia
November	Duitama, Colombia Haiphong, Vietnam

Since 1982, Operation Smile International has performed life-changing surgery on over 7,500 children outside the United States. Tens of thousands have been treated medically, and thousands of healthcare professionals have participated in an educational exchange.

In 1992, over 7,000 children in the United States received free medical care from Operation Smile.

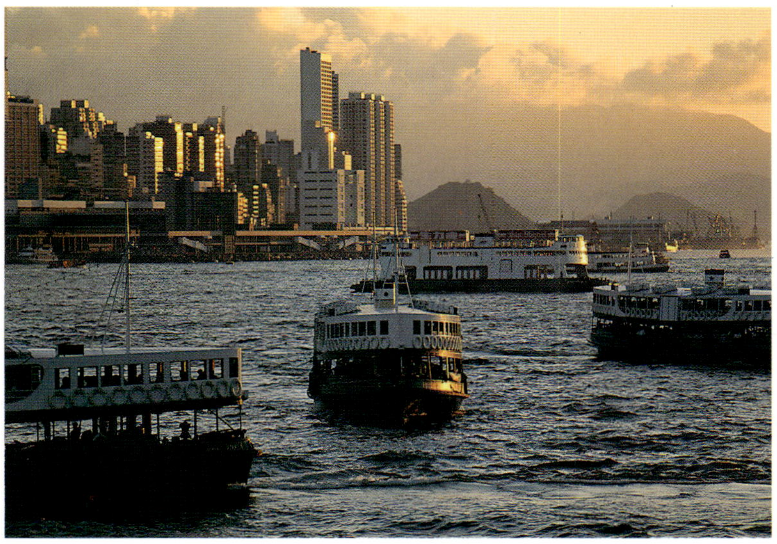

A special thanks to the supporters and volunteers of Operation Smile Hong Kong for backing the vision of this book, and specifically, Suzanna Hung for her efforts in guiding this project to completion.